Raphael

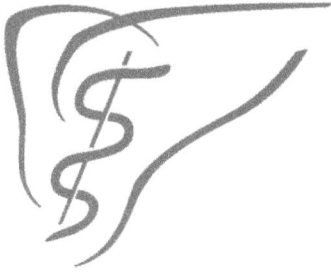

and the Mysteries of Illness and Healing

Material and motifs

collected by Michaela Glöckler

Medical Section at the Goetheanum

Contents

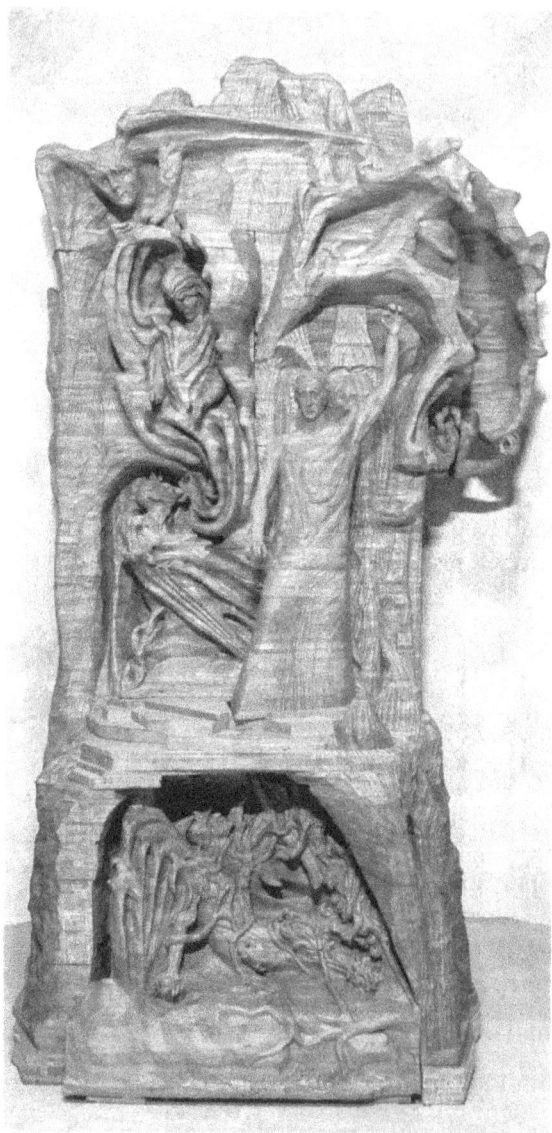

Sculpture, elm wood. Carved by Rudolf Steiner and Edith Maryon
between 1915 and 1924

Preface

When I took on the leadership of the Medical Section at the Goetheanum in 1988 I was often asked what the task of this section is. This motivated me to study again *The Christmas Conference for the Foundation of the General Anthroposophical Society 1923-1924*[1], as well as *Anthroposophical Leading Thoughts, Anthroposophy as a Path of Knowledge,* and *The Michael Mystery*[2] in relation to this question. There Rudolf Steiner describes the nature and task of the social framework set up by him. For medicine this means to develop the medical system of Anthroposophy and cultivate a professional community, i.e., the anthroposophic-medical movement. The latter is also sketched in principle in a way that goes straight to the heart in his *Curative Education Course,*[3] his pastoral-medical lectures[4] and his courses for young doctors[5] – but how can one encourage and develop such a task? Where are the colleagues and coworkers through whom it becomes possible? How can this succeed internationally?

Answers to these questions came through life and the concrete work itself in the section. Manifold forms of collaboration arose, enabling ever more activity in the Section – both at the Goetheanum and worldwide.

There were also guiding motifs that proved helpful. Especially the motif to connect the medical work and all of the therapies consciously and as much as possible to the source of knowledge from which this collaboration was inspired and which united Rudolf Steiner and Ita

---

[1] Rudolf Steiner: *The Christmas Conference for the Foundation of the General Anthroposophical Society 1923-1924.* Anthroposophic Press 1990 (vol. GA 260)

[2] Rudolf Steiner: *Anthroposophical Leading Thoughts. Anthroposophy as a Path of Knowledge. The Michael Mystery.* Rudolf Steiner Press 1999 (vol. GA 26)

[3] Rudolf Steiner: *Education for Special Needs. The Curative Education Course.* Rudolf Steiner Press 1999 (vol. GA 317)

[4] Rudolf Steiner: *Broken Vessels. The Spiritual Structure of Human Frailty.* Anthroposophic Press 2003 (vol. GA 318)

[5] Rudolf Steiner: *Course for Young Doctors.* Mercury Press 1997 (vol. GA 316)

Wegman. This was the collaboration that led to the inauguration of Anthroposophic Medicine and, in a completely new way, also to the question of Raphael as the archangel of the art of healing.

In recent years I have repeatedly encountered growing interest in this question concerning the being of Raphael, so I have decided to compile a few relevant motifs as a contribution to further discussion.

Michaela Glöckler
Medical Section at the Goetheanum
September 2015

Raphael – and the Mysteries of the Art of Healing

Raphael:

The sun intones, in ancient tourney
With brother spheres, a rival air;
And his predestinated journey,
He closes with a thunderous blare.
His sight, as none can comprehend it,
Gives strength to angels; the array
Of works, unfathomably splendid,
Is glorious as on the first day.

Beginning of Prologue in Heaven in Goethe's *Faust*[6]

Raphael is the archangel of the art of healing.

"Rapha" means physician in Hebrew. "EL" is the abbreviation of the name of the Elohim divinity in the biblical creation stories. We meet this archangel as the physician who accompanies and advises in the biblical legend of Tobias (see page 49 ff.). We also meet him in spirit in the book of Job, which bears witness to the causes of the world's most famous case of illness, the course of the illness and finally Job's successful healing. Raphael's name is not mentioned in the book of Job, but we find the "Raphaelic spirit" in it. Raphael is the spirit who sees the causes and effects of illnesses rooted in the spiritual development of the human being, and – out of this source – teaches the Mysteries of the healing arts. It is in this spirit that Goethe wrote his *Faust* – the drama of humanity for the fifth post-Atlantean cultural age that began according to Rudolf Steiner's spiritual-scientific research in the year 1413 and will continue until the year 3573. This epoch concerns the individualization of the human being, the gradual emancipation from familiar group connections such as those of folk, religion, social values, family and profession.

Goethe coined the epoch-making sentence:

Those who cannot give an account of the last three thousand years remain in the dark, living day by day, inexperienced.[7]

Rudolf Steiner goes even further. He spans his human consciousness from the Earth's origins as "old Saturn" to "Vulcan", the final incarnation of this planet and its inhabitants. Midway in this vast evolution he points

---

[6] Johann Wolfgang Goethe: *Faust*. Part I. The Harvard Classics. 1909-14.
[7] Johann Wolfgang Goethe: *West-östlicher Divan*. Berlin 1974

to a cultural connectedness, like a *cosmic Uterus*[8] He describes how each individual human life is embedded in the rhythms of the solar system. A human being breathes circa 18 times per minute when at rest. This means that he breathes 18 x 60 times per hour and per 24 hours 18 x 60 x 24 times = 25,920 times. This number corresponds to the famous "Platonic number" of the world-year, the time of the precession of the Spring equinox through the entire zodiac. This number marks the Mystery of the breath in the deepest sense, which is also the Mystery of Raphael.

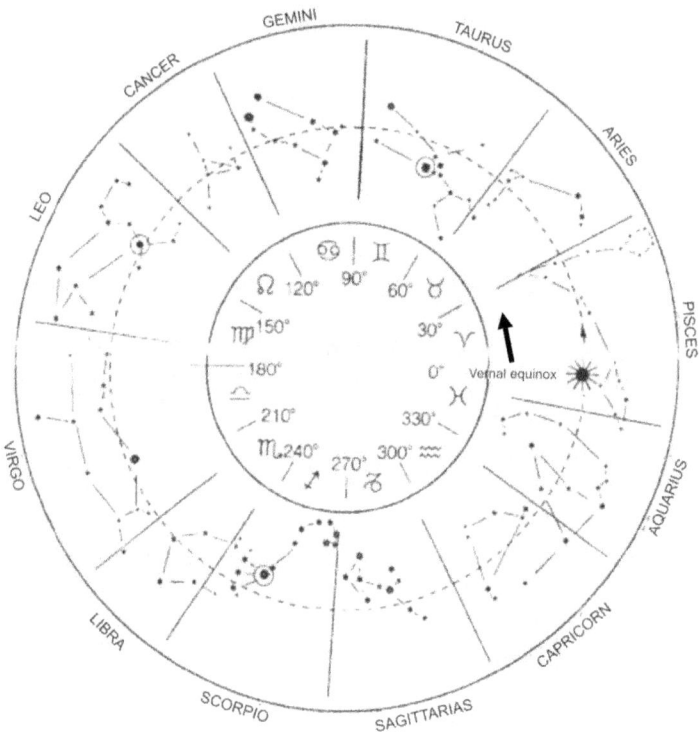

Diagram: The sun at the vernal equinox. The arrow shows its direction of movement through the zodiac, with the Earth at the center. The vernal equinox as such moves in the opposite direction, requiring approximately 25,920 years to go around the zodiac.

---

[8] Rudolf Steiner: *Broken Vessels. The Spiritual Structure of Human Frailty.* Anthroposophic Press 2003 (vol. GA 318), lecture of 17 Sept. 1924

It is interesting that the precession of the Earth's axis, as we know it from modern astronomy, is also related to this platonic number. The Earth turns one time around its own axis in approximately 24 hours; in 25,920 years its axis describes a complete circular cone.

Diagram: Precession of the Earth's axis. The Earth with its axis from North (N) to South (S), which moves as on the surface of a cone (arrow). The circle depicts the Earth with its axis.

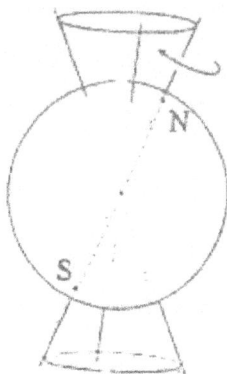

While the Earth's axis moves around a conic surface once every approximately 25,920 years, the Earth itself has moved approx. 25,920 times around the sun – in the opposite direction of the precession movement.

In terms of cultural history this time span of 25,920 years encompasses twelve cultural epochs: five Atlantean and seven post-Atlantean epochs, each averaging 2160 years. For the seven post-Atlantean epochs Rudolf Steiner indicated seven evolutionary Mysteries in his early esoteric lectures: [9]

for the ancient Indian epoch the Mystery of the Abyss,
for the ancient Persian epoch the Mystery of the Number,
for the Egypto-Chaldean-Babylonian-Assyrian epoch
    the Mystery of Alchemy,
for the Greco-Latin epoch the Mystery of the Death,
for the 5th cultural epoch the Mystery of Evil,
for the 6th cultural epoch the Mystery of the Word,
for the 7th cultural epoch the Mystery of Godliness.

If we let this sequence of evolutionary Mysteries work on us, we can recognize a common motif: the individualization of the human being.

[9] Rudolf Steiner: *An Esoteric Cosmology.* St. George Publications 1978 (vol. GA 94), lecture of 13 June 1906

Processes of Individualization in Human Evolution

In the ancient Indian epoch human beings learned to differentiate the world of the senses, the world of "Maya", from their trusted world of the spirit. For the first time they could use their senses consciously and individually.

In the ancient Persian epoch thinking became individualized. Numbers were discovered as purest thought and their ordering power was used.

In the Egyptian time of the pyramids, curative Medicine was heard of for the first time, as well as Alchemy as the secret of healing substances. On a soul level the life of feeling became individualized, especially through the experience of personal guilt and illness.

In the Greco-Latin epoch human will became individualized by facing the riddle of death: *The relics of my earthly sojourn are indestructible throughout the Æons of Time.* Goethe has his Faust speak these words at the end of his life. At the beginning of the modern age, Faust was already certain of what the evolutionary task of the fourth cultural epoch was, namely to grapple with the question of what remains after death. Not until we wished to remain connected with our individual deeds did individual continuity of the will become a fact of consciousness. Only then did the question become concrete of what will happen after life on earth to the person who performed the actions. The death of Christ on Golgotha answered this question for humanity.

In the fifth cultural epoch of humankind – our present era – it is all about individualizing our Ego. It is about the above mentioned separation from group connections of family, folk, tradition and culture. Those identity-giving group-forming forces are strong, which is why it is so difficult for each person to free himself from them and decide where and how to join with others to tackle specific tasks. The most difficult is to accomplish the transformation from being someone controlled and "educated" by societal norms and codes, laws and rules. When external control diminishes, and the will for autonomous self-determination is not yet ready to take over, all kinds of possibilities for error and power-abuse can emerge. These are the shadow sides inherent in developing an autonomous individual "I" in the fifth cultural epoch. The cultural Mystery of this current epoch is thus the appearance of inclinations towards evil. Therefore this question is important today: how can the battle wounds be healed that are caused by the Egoity freeing itself (see the macrocosmic Lord's Prayer on page 11) as it wrestles with its own evil inclinations and intentions? Here a "Raphaelic culture" is necessary, a coming together of many people with a will to orient, accompany, help and impart healing.

To understand something of the Mysteries of healing and to work with them in individual and social life is thus a core task of the fifth cultural epoch.

The sixth cultural epoch will be devoted to community-building out of the strength of the "I". The instrument for this is a new way of working with the word. The way in which it is presently used to impart information and clarify misunderstanding – or cause it – will not be its use in the future. The manner of speaking will make the speaker's intentions much more tangible, usage of the word will become an expression of the individual "I" and establish trust between individuals.

In the seventh epoch the individual will learn to connect consciously with the whole of humankind and will comprehend the meaning of creation and of human development. This comprehending and affirming of the individual human being, who is grateful to be allowed to develop himself – this is bliss for God and his hierarchies. They see their work as "done" and learn something new: the experiences of individual human beings on the challenging path of "I"-development.

These evolutionary Mysteries have the task of individualization in common: sense-perception, thinking, feeling and willing are abilities innately present in everyone as gifts of evolution, but in order to "own" them, we have to acquire them individually. However, this is most difficult with the human "I", the "self". How can we lose it, in order to find it anew completely out of ourselves? Rudolf Steiner puts this Mystery into words in one of his meditations within the framework of the esoteric school:

> In thinking awaken: you are in the spirit-light of the world.
> Experience yourself as radiant, *touching* the radiance.
>
> In feeling awaken: You are in the spirit-deeds of the world.
> Experience yourself, *feeling* spirit-deeds.
>
> In willing awaken: you are in the spirit-being of the world.
> Experience yourself, *thinking* spirit being.
>
> In the "I" awaken: you are in your own spirit-being.
> Experience yourself, *receiving* being from the Gods
> giving it to yourself.[10]

---

[10] Rudolf Steiner: *"Freemasonry" and Ritual Work. The Misraim Service. Texts and Documents from the Cognitive-Ritual Section of the Esoteric School 1904-1919.* SteinerBooks 2007 (vol. GA 265), Documents from new beginnings after World War I

The drama of the present situation of human development makes the difficulties connected with this task, as a kind of global identity crisis, abundantly clear. It is particularly shattering that evil in human nature is not "calculable", predictable, derivable directly from a person's education and development. Rather it is "banal", as Hannah Arendt[11] puts it, and can potentially be encountered in anyone. The abyss of evil must open as a possibility in every human being, with all the horrors and enticements of the "non I", so that step by step, out of our own experience, out of our own strength alone, we work our way through to the truth of our being.

Christian Morgenstern expressed this task of the fifth cultural epoch very aptly in one of his poems:

> *Those who walk to the truth*
> *they walk alone*
> *No one can be for the other*
> *on his path a brother.*
>
> *A short span it seems*
> *we go in choir ...*
> *until at last we see*
> *each one retires.*
>
> *Even the dearest one struggles*
> *somewhere afar,*
> *but who in total achieves it*
> *reaches a star,*
>
> *Creates his self enchristened,*
> *new god-filled ground – and*
> *is greeted by his brothers'*
> *eternal round.[12]*

Job's Story – Prototype of a Life Crisis

The Christian prophecy that everyone can reach freedom by knowing the truth, and that such a path will culminate in a community of "free spirits", gives a clear perspective and can help in overcoming different collective value systems in which social control and external directives lend protection against errors and "evil". What was good or bad used to be written in

---

[11] Hannah Arendt: *Eichmann in Jerusalem. A Report on the Banality of Evil.* Penguin Classics 2010

[12] Translated from Christian Morgenstern: *Wir fanden einen Pfad.* Zbinden Verlag 2014

laws, and was not the responsibility of the single individual. This only changed as a consequence of the spread of Christianity. Therefore it is quite astonishing to see that even before Christ's appearance on earth, this new direction sounds forth already in the book of Job, as if to prepare humanity for the future.

When reading the book of Job, we witness the fact that God punishes one who is loyal and righteous – against all previous tradition. We are shown a "good" person being tested. Everything he owns is taken from him – a situation resembling a severe life crisis – very familiar to all of us in today's world. What hails from the past does not support us anymore, and new prospects are not yet in sight. An extensive questioning begins, and protesting, as well as desperation. Job cannot comprehend it; neither can his relatives and friends. They believe that secretly he must suffer from a great sin. Job also doubts – himself and the justice of the world for which God stands. He has to rethink his relationship to God. Tradition had taught him that "God does not punish the just". He is not aware of any wrong-doing, any transgressions; he cannot understand himself nor the world anymore. Only when it becomes possible for him – stimulated by many conversations with people around him – to reconsider the identity of God completely out of himself, and to realize how superior God in His great perfection is compared to any human being – only when he sees God in all His works which include the potential for evil given to human beings, only when he recognizes that he is a part of a great and perfect wholeness, can he ask:

Shall mortal man be more just than God? shall a man be more pure than his maker? (Job 4:17)

Only when he sees himself before the countenance of God in the mirror of the good and perfect, can he feel:

Behold, happy is the man whom God correcteth: therefore despise not thou the chastening of the Almighty: (Job 5:17)

For he maketh sore, and bindeth up: he woundeth, and his hands make whole. (Job 5:18)

For, only in the face of perfection does Job experience his own "becoming", his evolving nature, and experiences deeply his lasting imperfection, and can say to God:

I will say unto God, Do not condemn me; shew me wherefore thou contendest with me. (Job 10:2)

He recognizes that he is in a process of development and needs instruction. He feels that the confrontation with evil, error and guilt cannot be absent from the path to perfection, that this is part of being human and it belongs to him. However, he also realizes that the wish to perfect his human nature is planted in his heart as a goal of evolution. Rudolf Steiner expressed this in a particularly urgent way especially in his *esoteric Lord's Prayer:*

> *Father, You who were, are, and will be in our inmost being!*
>
> *May your name be glorified and praised in us.*
>
> *May your kingdom grow in our deeds and inmost lives.*
>
> *May we perform your will as you, Father, lay it down in our inmost being.*
>
> *You give us spiritual nourishment, the bread of life, superabundantly in all the changing conditions of our lives.*
>
> *Let our mercy toward others make up for the sins done to our being.*
>
> *You do not allow the tempter to work in us beyond the capacity of our strength - for no temptation can live in your being, Father, and the tempter is only appearance and delusion, from which you lead us, Father, through the light of knowledge.*
>
> *May your power and glory work in us through all periods and ages of time.*[13]

Although this completeness is seeded in every human being's Selfhood as a spark of God, we incessantly incur guilt towards each other. We only appear to avoid piling up much guilt of our own. Do we not learn just as much from the errors of others as from our own? Do they not incur guilt also for our sakes, so that we do not need to? This fact, which Job recognized, exhorts us to turn to the macrocosmic Lord's Prayer, which Rudolf Steiner tells us was revealed to Jesus and spoken by him in a deserted temple after his baptism in the river Jordan. Jesus experiences the *sway of evil* on Earth with great compassion for human beings and he

---

[13] Rudolf Steiner: *Mantrische Sprüche. Seelenübungen II.* Rudolf Steiner Verlag 1999 (vol. GA 268), p. 341

recognizes that this *Selfhood guilt through others incurred* has to be in order for the individual person to become conscious of his own Selfhood. This requires also a period of detachment from God:

> *Amen*
> *The evils hold sway,*
> *Witness of egoity freeing itself.*
> *Selfhood guilt through others incurred,*
> *Experienced in the daily bread,*
> *Wherein the will of the heavens does not rule,*
> *Because man separated himself from your realm,*
> *And forgot your names,*
> *You Fathers in the heavens.*[14]

Sensing this, Job can accept his destiny and he asks for help for his further path, while admitting his own imperfection. His "guilt" consisted in the fact that he thought he had none...

Then Job answered the LORD, and said, I know that thou canst do every thing, and that no thought can be withholden from thee. Who is he that hideth counsel without knowledge? therefore have I uttered that I understood not; things too wonderful for me, which I knew not. Hear, I beseech thee, and I will speak: I will demand of thee, and declare thou unto me. I have heard of thee by the hearing of the ear: but now mine eye seeth thee. Wherefore I abhor myself, and repent in dust and ashes. (Job 42:1-6)

After this decisive step in self-knowledge born from deepest pain, his destiny can turn to the good again. He becomes healthy, his wealth returns and he reaches a great age.

The Raphaelic Signature in Goethe's *Faust*

Goethe opens his *Faust* with a prologue in heaven, beginning with the words of Raphael (see page 3). Raphael witnesses a bargain that God makes with the devil, giving him – as in the case of Job – permission to torment a righteous and striving human being such as Faust with all that is in the devil's power as long as he is here on earth. Here also the question of guilt as we normally understand guilt that awaits punishment, is not of interest. This is not what it is about. As with Job, it is really about the opposite: It is about a highly developed individual, agreeable to God. We

---

[14] Rudolf Steiner: *The Fifth Gospel*, Rudolf Steiner Press 2007 (vol. GA 148) p. 51

11

see here a human being ready for the next step in his development. The Lord is interested in what this human being can gain in his individual struggle with evil – it is not about punishment or judgment. Instead we hear "the Lord" speak these insightful words: *Man will err while yet he strives.* Raphael also does not present himself as a guardian of morality. Rather he is the one who is connected with the harmonies of the cosmos – the "brother spheres". He knows what unites and heals from inside. He knows of the strengthening power that proceeds from beholding the good, the true and the beautiful – and the perfect. He knows that the majestic and wholesome are stronger than the rage of destruction that plagues humanity on earth again and again, raising confusion as to the meaning of creation. The original "splendor", the knowledge about healing, the "strength" is his domain.

After the dialogue in heaven between God and the devil, Faust experiences something similar to Job, with him though, it shows on the soullevel not in bodily or outer suffering. For him too, everything becomes null and void that he appreciated before and he comes to the point where he has to say: *And thus existence is for me a weight,/ Death is desirable, and life I hate.*[15] Prior to this he had deplored:

> *And see that we can know – nothing!*
> *It almost sets my heart burning.*
> *I'm cleverer than all these teachers,*
> *Doctors, Masters, scribes, preachers:*
> *I'm not plagued by doubt or scruple,*
> *Scared by neither Hell nor Devil –*
> *Instead all Joy is snatched away,*
> *What's worth knowing, I can't say*
> *I can't say what I should teach*
> *To make men better or convert each.*
> *(...)*
> *Not even a dog would play this part!*

He needs a new identity, the past one has become useless, he desperately seeks a new one, right up to the edge of suicide. The one given by God and nature, also the one gained through academic studies and outer recognition does not sustain him anymore. Now he alone is challenged to achieve something, along his own paths of error and striving, to build a

---

[15] Johann Wolfgang Goethe: *Faust.* The Harvard Classics 1909-14, Study

new identity. Finding his path among the old traditions through exercise and schooling is not sufficient anymore. A decisive step is still lacking. He awakens to the school of destiny and to the *path of initiation through life* of which the Mystery of evil and the forces of destruction are also a part.

Rudolf Steiner comments in his *Philosophy of Spiritual Activity*:

> *Nature makes the human being a mere nature-being*
> *Society makes him one who acts lawfully*
> *Only he alone can make a free being out of himself.*[16]

The process of individualization of a human being happens through the experience of his very own personal destiny. In this, we are totally dependent on ourselves. Therefore Anthroposophy's impulse to make available to the individual the teaching of karma and reincarnation also clearly belongs to Raphael's sphere of working. To learn to identify with one's destiny, to recognize in it one's own individual path of development and to take on (co-)responsibility for it is a great challenge. Often it is only mastered with the help of therapeutic methods after experiencing illness and crises. Exemplary and prophetic for this future of humankind is the story of Tobias. It shows impressively how important a therapeutic companion can be.

To acquire knowledge, not only traditionally but on a path of self-experience, is not possible without error and guilt and the possibility of falling ill. That is why the school of Raphael is the school of life, "the path of initiation through life", where each one learns to retain health by way of understanding the laws of his own development. All learning from destiny serves the individualization and the return to health of the individual. Rudolf Steiner also refers to this as "hygienic occultism".[17]

Goethe makes this clear with Faust's visit to the witches' kitchen in his *Faust* Part 1. Here it is all about the drink of rejuvenation. Why does he show us the rejuvenation ceremony in the witches' kitchen? Faust is a man in the prime of life between 30 and 40 years old. At this age he does not actually need a rejuvenation potion to fall in love and seduce a woman. So, why is the Walpurgis Night brought into it? The Walpurgis

---

[16] Rudolf Steiner: *Intuitive Thinking as a Spiritual Path - A Philosophy of Freedom.* Anthroposophic Press 1995 (vol. GA 4), Chap. The Idea of Freedom
[17] Rudolf Steiner: *Die soziale Grundforderung unserer Zeit. In geänderter Zeitlage.* Rudolf Steiner Verlag 1990 (vol. GA 186), lecture of 1 Dec. 1918

Night leads us into realms where evil works magically. In contrast to the white magic of the Rosicrucians, here we get to know black magic. Goethe shows this to us in order to bring the dark side of human nature to our consciousness. The center of evil in the human being, the "caldron" or metabolic system, does not only have anabolic, regenerating forces but also catabolic, destructive forces in it. In the witches' kitchen we are made aware of how these metabolic forces – symbolized by the caldron – can also be misdirected. Then it becomes a place where illness can transition into health, and health into illness. It can also become a place where we are in danger of forgetting our mission and renouncing our own development; a place where impulses of regression, where pathological backwards development, i.e. becoming younger, can occur. A place in us where an unlived life can burst forth with passionate force, becoming active at the wrong time – with all the consequences for the destiny of those affected, that then must be healed again. But also a place showing the origins of every form of misuse of power.

Goethe shows how this can happen with the example of the witches' arithmetic. He shows how reversals are possible, how the goal of human development can become endangered, and how the good can end up in the wrong place. Something is done there which is the opposite of cosmic harmony – where above and below are balanced, where each force works in relation to the others in its right place – for the benefit of the whole. He also shows the possibility of going astray in a physiological-bodily sense, of deliberately manipulating the metabolism in order to comprehend the Mystery of how body and soul work upon each other. He shows the Mystery of evil in its connection to human nature and the metabolic blood system.

The witches' arithmetic begins with an appeal to human intelligence: *You must understand* (*Remember then*). Even black magic must be learned. Intelligence is not per se good or true – it is only the context in which it acts and the aims that it serves that make it a worthy endeavor or the servant of destructive impulses. At first glance we experience a bewildering game of numbers when the witch intones:

> *Remember then!*
> *Of One make Ten,*
> *The Two let be,*
> *Make even Three,*
> *There's wealth for thee.*
> *The Four pass o'er!*

Of Five and Six,
(The witch so speaks,)
Make Seven and Eight,
The thing is straight:
And Nine is One
And Ten is none--
This is the witch's one-time-one![18]

Ten is the so-called Tetraktys of Pythagoras, according to which the 10 is a very special number because it is the sum of 1+2+3+4. These four (tetra) numbers are at the same time the number of members of the human being and for that reason, 10 was always seen as the sacred number of the human being. It is all about becoming human.

Four is the sign for the four-fold physical body; it is the sacred four, the number of the four elements: The solid, liquid, gaseous and warmth. Warmth itself has no material properties, yet it controls the conditions of matter. Everything changes through a process of heating and the same through cooling. Four is also the number for the elemental worlds, with gnomes for the physical body, undines for the ether body, sylphs for the astral body and salamanders for the ego, for warmth. But they all have to work together in order for the physical body to develop.

Three is the number of the ether body, it is threefold. Life is a continual struggle for balance, a forming and shaping, a process. That is why the rhythmic activity of heart and lungs is balanced between the nerve-system and the metabolic-limb system. *a changing weaving, a glowing life,* as Faust says to the Earth-Spirit during the Easter night.

Two is the number of the astral body: The polarity of Yin and Yang, above and below, heavenly and earthly. Two souls are dwelling in my breast. Faust experiences the double nature of his astral body. His dark nature is incarnated, passionate in his body, the other rises forcibly in quest of rarified ancestral spheres, as Faust says to Wagner at the end of this Easter walk.

One brings everything together; it stands for our ego-organization. With these numbers, games are played in the witch's kitchen. *And two let go,* here we see a clear parting from the higher soul. Doubt and discord, everything that guides man toward a path of spirit is eliminated. The human being is to be returned to the state of a nature being, ruled by the

---

[18] Johann Wolfgang Goethe: *Faust.* The Harvard Classics. 1909-14, Scene 6, The Witches' Kitchen

15

forces of nature, a kind of conscious elemental being. *Take three again.* Rob the ether body of its developmental potential, enjoy life, live it up, end the threefold tension of thinking, feeling and willing. *Then you are rich.* Then you have everything, and you don't have to seek anymore. *From five and six, so says the witch, make seven and eight. That does the trick.* Development ceases. *And nine is one.* The 10 and the 1 as representatives of the origin and goal of man have been eliminated. Nine becomes one, not ten anymore. Nine is the new one. *And ten is none.* The ten and the one have disappeared. Human goals have been disbanded. Then nine is one. Now what is left of man is in the "soup" in the caldron of the witches' kitchen. It is still good enough for self-enjoyment, for experiencing the Walpurgis Night, but not anymore for self-directed transformation and development. In the Walpurgis Night the whole colorful landscape is then presented, indicating what is left of the human being when he refuses development and the individualization of his ego.

Faust does not fully understand what is happening – he remains awake though, and says to himself in this situation: *If only I do not forget myself.* He thinks he is still in charge of himself but notices that he is being "pushed". And he notices that it is about a black mass and about black magic. He experiences a strengthening of his self-confidence in the face of evil. Those who read *Faust* from a medical-therapeutic point of view experience the drama of all that harms and sickens. He also experiences which forces have to be called upon to heal the human being.

Here we become aware of the Raphael Mystery in artistic form. What is this Mystery of illness and healing? What is the secret of the Mercury staff? It is the secret of the power of the "I" to achieve an upright stance – in both body and spirit. It is the sign and the symbol for the ether body warmed through and guided by the "I", which works in polarity by day: as an "incarnated", enlivening force that keeps the body healthy and as "excarnated" body-free, active thought organism. This thought organism enables the like-wise excarnated "I"-organization to engage in conscious thought activity which also causes depletion and wearing down. During the night, on the other hand, the ether body works in unison as a regenerating organism of formative forces, taking into consideration the repercussions of the thought-life.

During the day   During the night

Conscious life of thought

Etheric body active free of the body

Unconscious life of the body

Body-oriented work of the etheric body

Unconscious, regenerating life of the body:

Body-oriented, uniform work of the etheric body

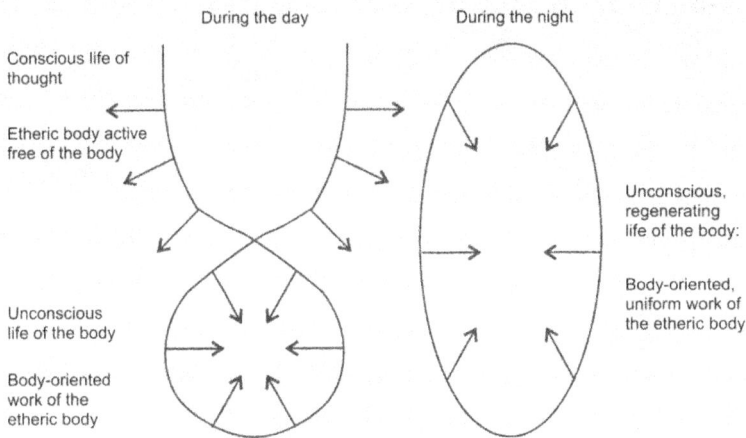

Diagram: If the ego was by day enthusiastically active in the thought-organism, warming it through, then it brings regenerating, life promoting after-effects from the thought-life into the nocturnal regenerative activity of the nervous system. If thinking was primarily oriented to the outer life-conditions, then it carries the after-effects of a thinking only attached to the world of physical existence.[19]

Happening night after night, the after-effects of our thought-life can work in an enlivening and ordering way on the organism's vitality, or else have a fixating, laming, chaotic effect on the processes of regeneration. Depending on the destiny situation, on the constitution and the life circumstances, this will bring necessary, additional strengthening to a person who needs this for his daily life, or it leads to a "karmic illness". What Goethe describes in the picture of the witches' kitchen and has his Faust experience, is what happens when the conceptual forces and the execution of life are not in harmony with one another and therefore harm the human being in body or soul. He describes the Mystery of the Mercury staff that encompasses the secret of the aberrations that are spoken of in the witch's arithmetic, as well as the effective connections from which all recovery proceeds.

---

[19] Rudolf Steiner and Ita Wegman: *Fundamentals of Therapy - An Extension of the Art of Healing through Spiritual-Scientific Knowledge*. Mercury Press 2010 (vol. GA 27), Chap. I

Raphael's Activity as an Easter Imagination

In autumn of 1923 Rudolf Steiner describes this Raphael-Mercury-Mystery in a comprehensive way in his Easter Imagination.[20] He presents how the course of the year is the archetypal picture of every healing process. The one-sidedness and with it the possibility of illness that may occur at one time of the year is balanced by another. He points out how in the solid and fluid elements Ahrimanic forces are at work and Luciferic forces are found in air and warmth. He makes very clear how the divine father-forces working in the natural order ever again establish new harmony to ensure a healthy balance. In the human being, however, this creative natural order is only working in the nature-bestowed bodily part. There the "devils", working in nature in a one-sided way (the Luciferic and Ahrimanic forces), are only balanced in the unconscious part of the human being, where his members are incarnated. In the conscious life of thought and in the consciously guided will and feeling-life, however, where the members of the human being work in an excarnated way, they need to be guided by the human being himself. There he is released into his personal responsibility and is therefore seducible into any kind of one-sidedness.

Such one-sidedness can become fixed and the balance can be obstructed. Here the human being himself must consciously establish the harmony, guiding and directing his development, affirming the fact of his many possibilities for error. In this, Christ is the great helper. Christ lives united with man as "Lord of the elements", and "Lord of karma". He maintains the "book of life" in which every "striving effort" is written. He does not judge but helps and "saves". In this Raphael, the "Christian Mercury" is His messenger, the inspirer of the community of physicians and therapists working together in this sense:

But now that man has advanced in freedom, he should use his freedom to banish the threatening danger that Ahriman will fetter him to the Earth. For in the perspective of the future this threat stands before him. And here we see how into Earth-evolution there came an objective fact: the Mystery of Golgotha.

Although the Mystery of Golgotha had indeed to enter as a one-time event into the history of the Earth, it is in a sense renewed for human beings every year. We can develop a feeling for how the Luciferic force up above would like to suffocate physical humanity in carbonic vapour, while down below, the Ahrimanic forces would like to vivify the limestone

---

[20] Rudolf Steiner: *The Four Seasons and the Archangels*. Rudolf Steiner Press 2002 (vol. GA 229), lecture of 7 October 1923

masses of the Earth with an astral rain, so that man himself would be calcified and reduced to limestone. But then, for a person who can see into these things, there arises between the Luciferic and the Ahrimanic forces the figure of Christ; the Christ who, freeing Himself from the weight of matter, has Ahriman under his feet; who wrested Himself free from the Ahrimanic and takes no heed of it, having overcome it, as is portrayed here [in the Goetheanum, MG] in painting and sculpture. And here is shown also how the Christ overcomes the force that seeks to draw the upper part of man away from the Earth. The head of the Christ-figure, the conqueror of Ahriman, appears with a countenance, a look and a bearing such that the dissolvent forces of Lucifer cannot touch them. The Luciferic power drawn into the earthly and held there – such is the form of the Christ as He appears every year in Spring. That is how we must picture Him: standing on earthly matter, which Ahriman seeks to make his own; victorious over death; ascending from the grave as the Risen One to the transfiguration which comes from carrying over the Luciferic into the earthly beauty of the countenance of Christ.

So there appears before our eyes, between the Luciferic and the Ahrimanic forms, the Risen Christ in his resurrected form as the Easter picture; the Risen Christ, with Luciferic powers hovering above and Ahrimanic powers under His feet.

(...)

But a completion in some form will be necessary if one is to grasp the whole idea. For all that can be seen as the threatening Luciferic influence and the threatening Ahrimanic influence belongs to the inner being of the Nature-forces and the direction they strive to take in spring and on into summer; and standing over against them is the healing principle that rays out from the Christ. But a living feeling for all this will be attained when the whole architectural scheme is completed and what I have described exists in architectural and sculptured form, and when in the future it will be possible to present in front of the sculpture a living drama with two leading characters - man and Raphael.

Within this architecture, and in the presence of the sculpture, there would have to be enacted a kind of Mystery Play, with man and Raphael as the chief characters – Raphael with the staff of Mercury and all that belongs to it. In living artistic work everything is a challenge, and fundamentally there is no sculpture and no architecture which – if it is to be inwardly in accord with cosmic truth – does not call for a presentation in the space surrounding it of the artistic action it embodies. At Easter this architecture and sculpture would call for a Mystery Play, showing man

19

taught by Raphael to see how far the Ahrimanic and Luciferic forces make him ill, and how through the power of Raphael he can be led to perceive and recognize the healing principle, the great world-therapy, which lives in the Christ-principle. If all this could be done – and the Goetheanum was designed for all of it – then at Easter there would be, amid much else, a certain culmination of all that can flow into mankind from the Ahrimanic and Luciferic secrets.

(...)

The presence of the World-Healer is felt: the Saviour who willed to lift the great evil from the world. His presence is felt. For in truth He was, as I have often said, the Great Physician in the evolution of mankind. This will be felt, and to Him will sacrifice be offered with all the wisdom about healing influences that man can possess. This would be included in the Easter Mystery, the Easter ritual; and by celebrating the Easter festival in this way we should be placing it quite naturally in the context of the seasonal course of the year.

(...)

All that can be learnt in this way under the influence of the great teacher Raphael – who is really Mercury in Christian terminology and in Christian usage should carry the staff of Mercury – can only reach its worthy culmination when it can become integrated into, and part of, the Easter ritual. Much else can come into them; of this I will speak in later lectures.[21]

The Harmonizing Force of Karma and the School of Raphael

The more people begin to understand their life in the sense of hygienic occultism, as an individual path of knowledge, the stronger the healing power for social working will be. When destiny relations harmonize, they become a support and make far-reaching tasks possible. This was the case to the highest degree between Rudolf Steiner and his doctor colleague Ita Wegman.[22,23] Raphael could therefore reveal himself in their collaboration. As a result the foundation for Anthroposophic Medicine was laid.

---

[21] Rudolf Steiner: *The Four Seasons and the Archangels*. Rudolf Steiner Press 2002 (vol. GA 229),, lecture of 7 October 1923

[22] J. Emanuel Zeylmans van Emmichoven: *Die Erkraftung des Herzens: Eine Mysterienschulung der Gegenwart. Rudolf Steiners Anleitungen für Ita Wegman*. Ita Wegman Institut 2009

[23] Margarete und Erich Kirchner-Bockholt: *Die Menschheitsaufgabe Rudolf Steiners und Ita Wegman*. Philosophisch-Anthroposophischer Verlag 1976

Its goal is to promote individual health in the context of a social framework. This "primal" health is rooted in the "I" of man that wishes to recognize himself and the meaning of his existence. Raphael accompanies this as the teacher.

When Ernst Lehrs, a Waldorf teacher of the first hour and author of the work *Man or Matter* asked Rudolf Steiner how we could recognize the being of Raphael in contrast to Michael about whom we can read so much in Anthroposophy, he answered: *the path to Michael is relatively easy in our time. Then for a long time there is nothing – and only then – – – the being of Raphael.*

I learned of these indications from Ernst Lehrs himself during the time of my university studies. I asked myself again and again: did Rudolf Steiner simply want to give this answer to the highly gifted mathematician and natural scientist to get him to "think for himself"? He belonged to the group of young people who had asked Steiner for the youth course[24], where Michael the Spirit of our Time is central. Or was Steiner's answer to him: *You still have a long time to work with the Michael-knowledge; do not ask already for the next work project!* The answer can also be taken quite literally to be the truth, that it is a long path that leads from thought and felt insight to personal life experience and realization. Is it not this, the long path that leads from the head through the heart to the hand, and into the metabolism that strengthens the hand, the path from Michael to Raphael? The good can only be found when we do it. As long as we merely think and feel it, it is not there. The meditation that Rudolf Steiner gave to young doctors and medical students would, in this respect, be the central Raphael meditation. It is titled: How do I find the Good?[25] In this lecture about hygienic occultism, Rudolf Steiner described life itself as being analogous to the process of becoming ill that continually needs healing. And he adds to this picture the mercurial wisdom of the dual nature of the etheric as a healing life force on the one hand and as thinking, knowing, on the other. Whereby the healing power in the organism corresponds to true, spiritually enlightened knowledge: *The innate healing power of the human organism transformed into knowledge results in occult knowledge.*[26]

---

[24] Rudolf Steiner: *Becoming the Archangel Michael's Companions.* SteinerBooks 2007 (vol. GA 217)

[25] See also Peter Selg: *Die "Wärme-Meditation": Geschichtlicher Hintergrund und ideelle Beziehungen.* Verlag am Goetheanum 2013

[26] Rudolf Steiner: *Die soziale Grundforderung unserer Zeit In geänderter Zeitlage.* Rudolf Steiner Verlag 1990 (vol. GA 186), lecture of 1 Dec. 1918

As a medical student I asked Rita Leroi,[27] the oncologist and long-term director of the Lukas Clinic in Arlesheim, how it might be possible to connect with the Archangel Raphael. She answered: Michael is the countenance of Christ – Raphael His helping hand. He lives in the doctor-patient-relationship, *where two or more are gathered in my name*. He is a brotherly companion, advisor and helper in need. He embodies the essence of selfless aid and service for others.

I was full of enthusiasm when I heard that together with the esoteric founding of the Medical Section at the Goetheanum in September 1924, the beginning of a Raphael school was also intended. It could only be established in seed form, and still waits to be developed. Rudolf Steiner's indications point on one hand in the direction of karma-knowledge as the school of life and development. On the other hand, they guide doctors and pharmacists on a path to understand the nature of substances and their medical benefits for the individual human being and for typical illness-processes. Rudolf Steiner offers a clear seminal characterization of this impulse for a Raphael School in the pastoral-medical mantram, a direction-giving meditation that he formulated at the end of his joint course for doctors and priests.

> *I will go the path,*
> *Which dissolves the elements into process*
> *And leads me downwards to the Father*
> *Who sends the illness as balance to karma.*
> *And leads me upwards to the Spirit*
> *Who guides the soul in error to attainment of freedom.*
> *Christ leads downwards and upwards*
> > *Harmoniously creating Spirit-Man in earthly man.*[28]

But we receive the most comprehensive teaching about this new school wisdom through the explanations in the book written together with Ita Wegman, *Fundamentals of Therapy.*[29] The first seven chapters are

---

[27] Silke Helwig: *'Es geht um mein Leben': Zum 100. Geburtstag von Rita Leroi.* Zbinden Verlag 2013

[28] Rudolf Steiner in: *The Anthroposophic-Medical Movement. Responsibility Structures and Modes of Work.* Verlag am Goetheanum 2010, p. 125, also in *Broken Structures. The Spiritual Structure of Human Frailty.* Anthroposophic Press 2003 (vol. GA 318)

[29] Rudolf Steiner and Ita Wegman: *Fundamentals of Therapy - An Extension of the Art of Healing through Spiritual-Scientific Knowledge.* Mercury Press 2010 (vol. GA 27)

dedicated to health – to the relationship between the healthy human microcosm and the macrocosm.

The first chapter reveals the Mystery of the Mercury staff: the metamorphosis of growth forces into thinking forces (see page 47 ff.).

The second chapter gives a thorough explanation of how illness can arise when the human being is active in soul and spirit and falls into one-sidedness and error.

The third to fifth chapters introduce the microcosmic and macrocosmic nature of the members of the human being and their specific configuration of forces. They also describe in a moving way what sacrifices and what experiences the now earthly substances suffer. And how this sacrifice finds its deliverance and fulfilment when the substance can become "spirit bearing" in the human being.

The sixth chapter portrays the embryonic development of the human body in such a way that one can learn to think the physiological processes of the working members of the human being and to picture the formation of the various organs.

The seventh chapter describes the entire healthy organism as one open for development and not closed off within itself, showing the nature of self-destructive and self-healing forces.

Chapters eight to twelve then serve to describe the five central causes that lead to metabolic illnesses. These are illustrated by means of the working of sugar, protein, fat, uric acid and warmth. The members of the human being as they regulate the metabolic processes become evident in their physical and soul activity.

Five therapy chapters follow, which focus on the therapeutic regulation of the relationship between the ether and astral bodies, then the regulating power of the "I"-organization, then the possible weakening of the physical-etheric constitution in the course of ageing, the principle of finding remedies, and an introduction to understanding substances as a foundation for understanding remedies.

The last three chapters of the book are devoted to the working principles of eurythmy therapy, a demonstration of the practice of Anthroposophic Medicine by means of nine clinical examples, and the use of typical medicines that have been developed to address certain typical illnesses.

This is the fundamental course, and – as Ita Wegman writes in her unpublished preface to this book – *the correct reading of this book will make it possible for every doctor to behold the illnesses himself spiritually.*

23

Illness as unconscious Initiation Event

The cited texts and motifs of Raphaelic wisdom have one thing in common: They describe the mercurial dynamic that leads the upper forces – the excarnated cognitive life – into the realm of the lower forces – the unconscious life of the metabolism, and vice versa. This work dynamic is thus also identical to the threshold drama that is enacted between the world of the senses and the supersensible world. It shows how illness can arise because at the crossing of this threshold to the spiritual world, in body, soul and sprit – for whatever reason – the right orientation is lost. However, it is decisive here that illness is not branded as flaw, mistake or error. Rather, it seems that the meaning of an illness is its manifestation itself because it brings – even if painful – correction so that healing can begin. Seen spiritually in this way, illness appears as something good – which creates a place in the body or soul where the necessary compensation of destiny can take place. It appears as something that the person evidently needs for his "salvation", something he wants to go through – but cannot achieve in a healthy way at the "right time and place". Now his personal, social or human destiny gives him the opportunity to acquire this experience through illness. This was not achieved in a conscious way, on a path of knowledge – inspired by Michael – but unconsciously through pain and suffering accompanied by Raphael.

Rudolf Steiner writes in his notebook when preparing for the course for young doctors:

At the threshold stream
Senses' dark and spirit's light
Into each other, creating illusion.

Illness is the reflection of this illusion
In illness lives the Guardian:

Encounter conscious in spirit,
Encounter unconscious in body.[30]

---

[30] Rudolf Steiner in: *The Anthroposophic-Medical Movement. Responsibility Structures and Modes of Work.* Verlag am Goetheanum 2010, p. 22, also in Rudolf Steiner: *Mantrische Sprüche. Seelenübungen II. 1903-1925.* Rudolf Steiner Verlag 1999 (vol. GA 268). Notebook, January 1924, p. 304

The Question for a Renewal of the Medical Mysteries

It was Ita Wegman who asked Rudolf Steiner directly about the Raphael Mystery – that is, about new Christian Mysteries of healing.

In the second volume of the biographical work *Who was Ita Wegman* we find a notebook entry by Ita Wegman in connection with a medical conference in Arlesheim, October 1936, that contains her own record of her question and Rudolf Steiner's answer:

I posed two questions to Rudolf Steiner; I can give the exact time when they were posed. The first question in England after the Summer school in Penmaenmawr: Why is the Mystery aspect of Medicine not placed into the foreground anymore and cast into a form? Why are the medical courses given so intellectually? It has to be that way, Rudolf Steiner answered, because the conditions to work differently are not here yet. That you pose this question though is essential. In October/November 1923, he then gave the many Mystery lectures, the Michael, Christmas, Easter, St. John's Imaginations, in which he brought the cosmic healing arts. The Christmas Conference was founded, new life sprouted into the Anthroposophical Society. There was really a beginning to fashion the medical work differently. I remind you of the lectures given to the young doctors. The Mystery principle is that we learn to think in pictures, that the events of the whole universe are taken up in pictures, including healing in the cosmos and healing in the microcosm, which is only a picture of the macrocosm. The pictures then have to be gathered together into meditations.

My second question to Rudolf Steiner was shortly before his illness, in September 1924. I asked: Is it possible to found a medical Mystery school?

Rudolf Steiner's answer was: This cannot so easily be done, it has to be wanted by the spiritual world and there have to be people who want to receive it.

After a few days he said to me that he had asked the Mercury-Raphael spirit and had received a confirming answer. He was given the task to renew an old custom that formerly took place in the holy, old sanctuaries, under the guidance of Mercury-Raphael. I received the task to seek human souls who aspire toward the spirit, and have an inner wish for such work and want to listen to the words of Raphael.

Following this, we made a very small beginning. In this way a seed was planted for a Raphael school.

My dear friends this was significant. To bring together the healing principles that lived in the different Mysteries to be gathered in one school. Michael and Raphael working together!

Regretfully, it was not to be. We literally felt the resistance of the earth. Earth and humans did not yet want such a powerful spirituality. Dr. Steiner then left his earthly work voluntarily, for his illness was only Maya. And human beings were left alone, and fell back into old habits of judging everything intellectually and only out of reason. The Anthroposophical Society was shaken to its foundations, karmic connections became confused. Humans did not yet have the maturity to receive so much spirituality, or, to look at the positive in conflict and strife, sensing that the maturity was not yet there, retarding forces – often necessary – resisted the course of events to preclude spiritual imperfections from spiritual evolution. This is how it looks.

We long for a Mystery medicine. We cannot just continue what was begun. We must try to prepare ourselves again to awaken a Spirit recalling in us of all that the old Mysteries once were. I will do whatever is in my power to do so.

Clarify who the being of Mercury-Raphael really is.

Michael assists the human being in his battle to change nature-consciousness into self-consciousness, and to establish it. Michael is present, the spiritual, cosmic healer, working on the head, while Raphael-Mercury stands next to man working into his breathing system. The flaming sword of Michael is cast out of cosmic iron and with this force Michael battles the nature consciousness that wants to rise in man, in order to draw out the consciousness of the self. (Notebook 57)[31]

Nine years before, in 1927, at one of the first larger medical conferences after Rudolf Steiner's death, Ita Wegman presented her situation as leader of the Medical Section in this way: *It became necessary for me to represent Rudolf Steiner's method which was for me, obviously, a matter of course, but it was, on the other hand also not possible for me to predict how far I would succeed in this. Time was needed to grow into the method, time also to let this method of healing ripen, in order to stand on one's own feet and move forward. Many difficulties that presented themselves in the Society also did not make it easy for the Medical Section. It could not immediately do justice to all the demands that were addressed to it. For example, it could at first not work scientifically in outer life, in the sense that was necessary and demanded. So, for a longer time, the work was more preparatory, in order to gather experiences, in order to grasp with a deeper understanding all the indications that Dr. Steiner had given*

---

[31] J. E. Zeylmans-van Emmichoven: *Who Was Ita Wegman*, Vol. 2, Mercury Press 1995, p. 216-217 of the German edition

for the healing of illnesses. It was, at first, all about healing, and about gaining the conviction that with the experiences made, a basis could be created, on which the work could be carried to the outside.

Everywhere work was done and as far as possible experiences were exchanged and collected. In this way we gradually obtained a better overview and the shortcomings that were there could be recognized and improved. This again gave us the reason to examine experimentally, to find, on the one hand what the causes of the shortcomings were, and on the other to reinforce what Dr. Steiner put as facts before us from his scientific research. At the same time, a beginning was to be made for an activity reaching the outside. The outside world also gradually became aware of us through our successes in healing, and it demanded information and orientation. Due to this, the moment has come that demands of us to gather and consolidate the work more than before, in order to be prepared for all the demands placed on us by the outside world ... [32]

Mysteries of Wisdom, Mysteries of Will

We know about the old pre-Christian mysteries (as for instance the Egypto-Babylonian, those of Samothrace, of Greece and Hibernia) through Rudolf Steiner's descriptions[33] but also through historical documentation. These Mystery centers directed and ordered the cultural, political and practical life of the people. The awakening to historical and philosophical consciousness in the eighth century B.C. went hand in hand with the receding into decadence of the Mysteries, followed by their closing. A secularization and "de-spiritualization" of science began. Democratic, republican and anarchistic efforts then appeared. The prophecy of the Gospel of St. John began to fulfill itself more and more, which is true not only for elite rulers but for every single human being: *You will know the truth, and the truth will set you free.* (John 8:32) The most intimate secrets of the old Mysteries were thereby made public: the path of knowledge towards truth and towards the achievement of individual freedom of every single human being. The inscription on the temple of Apollo in Delphi reads: *Know yourself as a human being.* Another one reads: *Nothing too much*, which means: *Measure is all.* These two promptings, to know yourself as a human being and to find the middle path between all extremes was essentially the central teaching proceeding from the old

---

[32] ibid, p. 171-172 of the German edition
[33] Rudolf Steiner: *Mystery Knowledge and Mystery Centres.* Rudolf Steiner Press 1973 (vol. GA 232)

mysteries. Gradually, this teaching became a possession of the general culture. What then could be meant by a "renewal of the Mysteries"?

Is it not that people have now taken their destiny into their own hands and do they not choose for themselves who should take on the task of leadership in their community or state? Certainly, a renewal of the Mystery culture cannot go back to old forms of spiritual superiority or secret knowledge. Both were used to dominate the ignorant. Also the creation of a new secret elite would not signify an advance but rather a step backwards and would ignore the fact that Christ appeared on earth. The new Mysteries must respect the individualizing, unsure, error-prone human "I" and support it to find "itself". Only from a freed human "I" can the new Mysteries proceed, when many individuals begin to become more interested in the great affairs of humanity and become conscious out of their own initiative of their co-responsibility for the whole. The new Mysteries are Mysteries of will, Mysteries of the forming and shaping of the social life. Underlying this is the free decision of the individual human being who wishes to place his will into the service of others and the whole community.

The philosopher Johann Gottlieb Fichte (1762-1814) arrived at the following formulation: *The human being can do what he should do; and if he says: I cannot, he does not want to.* "Renewed" Mysteries in this sense are "Christian Mysteries". They carry on from the Christ Event, which Rudolf Steiner repeatedly spoke of as the Mystery of Golgotha or the Christ Event. The "Imitation of Christ" knows no know-it-alls, no seeking after outer influence or power plays. It only knows to address, to invite the will of the human being, in fact only the f r e e will. We can already see that this is the case in specifically Christian challenges:

Love your enemies, bless them that curse you, do good to them that hate you, and pray for them which despitefully use you, and persecute you, and pray for those who persecute you. (Matthew 5:44) One can only follow such appeals freely – it cannot be done out of duty or fear.

Rudolf Steiner elaborated on this in a public lecture on the Apocalypse of St John: *The more individualized a man becomes the more he can become a bearer of Love. Where the blood links men together they love because they are led to what they should love. When man is granted individuality, when he tends and nurtures the divine spark within him, then the impulses of love, the waves of love, pass from man to man out of the free heart. And thus with this new impulse man has enriched the old bond of love that is bound to the blood-tie. Love passes over gradually into*

spiritual love which flows from soul to soul and which will ultimately en-
compass all humanity in a common bond of brother-love. (...) Earlier
initiation was directed to times past, to age-old wisdom; Christian initia-
tion reveals the future to one who is to be initiated. That is a necessity;
man is to be initiated not only in wisdom, or in feelings but in his will.
For then he knows what he is to do, he can set himself a goal for the
future. Ordinary everyday people set themselves aims for the afternoon,
for the evening or the morning. The spiritual man is able, out of spiritual
principles, to set himself distant aims which pulse through his will and
make his forces quicken. To set goals before humanity means in the true,
highest sense, in the sense of the original Christ principle, to grasp Chris-
tianity esoterically. In this way it was grasped by the one who wrote the
great principle of the initiation of the will – the writer of the Apocalypse.
We misunderstand the Apocalypse, if we do not understand it as the im-
pulse given for the future, for action and deed.[34]

In describing these new Christian Mysteries that will lead humanity
into a future worthy of human beings, Rudolf Steiner could link them to
Goethe and, in particular, to Goethe's Fairy Tale. Here the Mystery
phrase for the future is heard when the old man with the lamp says: *A*
single person does not help, only one who unites himself with many others
at the right time.[35] The individuality, the single person – which was the
goal of development of the old Mysteries, right up to the birth of the ego
at the Mystery of Golgotha – now requires a new developmental motif.
While the folk and family communities of the past were led by individual
leaders, the new communities have to arise through many coming together at the "right time". Important happenings depend on whether the
leader necessary for them is successfully chosen, or accepted as a given,
necessary for something to succeed. It depends on the – "free" – will of
each person whether the "good" can occur. Whoever grasps this new sacred Mystery motif can understand why it was of such importance to
Rudolf Steiner from 1902 onwards when he took over the German section
of the Theosophical Society to inaugurate and nurture forms of community building. Even if some things did not succeed – such as the attempt

---

[34] Rudolf Steiner: *The Apocalypse of St. John.* Kessinger Publishing 2010 (vol. GA
104), Lecture of 17 June 1908 in Nuremburg
[35] Johann Wolfgang Goethe: *The Green Snake and the Beautiful Lily.* SteinerBooks
2006

to found a society for the theosophical way of life and art,[36] – it never prevented him from continuing to work in this direction. Ever more people came to him who were looking for indications and help in the renewal of the different professional fields of work, and as they did so the new professional ideals – for education, medicine, nursing, curative education, priesthood, agriculture, artistic activities and scientific striving – had a community-building effect in that people of a particular professional group united themselves with these new professional ideals and wanted to manifest the necessary social and societal communities in the sense of the new Mysteries. At least this was attempted.

On the Path to a New Mystery Culture

As we are stand with these attempts at the beginning of realizing a new Mystery culture, and have great difficulty individually as well as socially to understand what it is all about, we need orientation. This we can receive from studying the personalities who have already grasped this impulse, and have taken it up and as far as possible made it a reality. After Rudolf Steiner, the first such personalities were his three closest co-workers, Marie Steiner, Edith Marion and Ita Wegman. Already at the beginning of the century, Marie Steiner posed the question about the specifically Christian esoteric path of schooling for the Occident. She became the co-founder and nurturer of the whole anthroposophic work as the foundation of the Christian Mysteries. Edith Marion had in an exemplary way the bearing and character of a pupil and co-worker of these Mysteries in the field of the visual arts. Ita Wegman was the one who could ask very concretely about the renewal of the Mysteries in medicine. This was the decisive question that prompted Rudolf Steiner at Christmas 1923/24 to undertake the new founding of the Anthroposophical Society and the School of Spiritual Science, as an open esoteric Mystery school. She felt that the new Mystery is the Mystery of the individual deed and saw clearly that a humane medicine could only be developed on such a Mystery foundation.

In 1932 medical students asked the question: "What can the future still offer us?" Ita Wegman answered: *"We can put the question quite differently, we can ask: How can I form the future?"*

---

[36] See Rudolf Steiner: *From the History and Contents of the First Section of the Esoteric School 1904-1914*. Lecture of 15 December 1911 in Berlin (morning). SteinerBooks 2007 (vol. GA 264)

With this answer – that we should not ask what the future holds in store for us, but rather how can we form the future – Ita Wegman showed herself to be working in full consciousness within the will-stream of the sacred Mysteries, renewed by Christianity, also after the death of Rudolf Steiner. She stands before us as a human being who has completed the transition from the old to the new sacred Mysteries out of deep, inner insight and who lived and worked accordingly throughout the rest of her life. Nowadays the main task cannot be to demand more and more new knowledge, although it is welcome when new knowledge shows itself through diligence and exact research. Something else though, is necessary for the new Mysteries and must become part of our culture: to do what one knows. Humanity "knows" already far more than what it can cultivate or implement. It is rather our task to realize and make fruitful for development a small portion of what is already available as insight and knowledge. The nature of the new Mysteries consists in active doing, in manifesting wisdom that is individually recognized, penetrating it with feeling, that will transition into loved action. Rudolf Steiner describes this for our epoch in his lectures on the Apocalypse of St. John.

In reading the Apocalypse, one is shattered by the immense visions of evil, the horrors of human nature's bestial outbreaks that at first seem to be so irreconcilable with the revelation of the Christ Principle. And it is exactly this that points to the Mysteries of will. For will is based on the activity of the metabolism of the human being, and the secret of illness, of destruction, of evil is as much at the bottom of it as the forces of healing and regeneration. It belongs to the deepest riddles of Christianity that the Passion is part of the Mystery of Golgotha, which means torture, martyrdom and violent death accompanied by hate, mockery and derision – all expressions of the evil possibilities in human nature are part of it.

This riddle can only be resolved if we recognize in the ego-nature of human beings the double-edged sword of which the Apocalypse speaks.[37] This double-edge is connected with the ego's capacity for freedom: For one thing, the ego on its path of individualization has to separate itself from all that is familiar and become "itself". For the other, it has the possibility freely to unite itself again, to identify itself. In addition, it always has to decide anew and with presence of mind between two possibilities so that a middle path can become visible between caprice and compulsion, pride and self-sacrifice, waste and stinginess, foolhardiness and cowardice etc., accommodating one's own interests and those of one's

---

[37] *Revelation (Apocalypse)* 1:16

social surroundings. It is not a choice between good and evil but rather a continuous struggle for a state of balance between two extremes, Luciferic evil and Ahrimanic evil, they only work in an "evil" way as long as they experience no healing balance.[38] And so we should not be astonished that all the possibilities of aberration and horror which will still arise during the course of evolution of humanity as a consequence of ego endowment are already anticipated pictorially in the apocalyptic descriptions. They should not lead us to despair but rather fire our will, our decision to be ready to act in such a way as to serve the good.[39] In Rudolf Steiner's lecture of June 25th, 1908, in the cycle *The Apocalypse of St. John*, he says:

True Anthroposophy can only put forward as the final goal, a community of free and independent egos that have become individualized. It is just this that is the mission of the earth, which is expressed in love - that egos learn to confront one another freely. Love is not perfect if it proceeds from coercion, from people being chained together, but only when each "I" is so free and independent that it does not have to love, when its love is an entirely free gift. It is the divine plan to make this "I" so independent that as an individual being, in all freedom, it can offer love even to God. It would amount to man being led by the apron-strings of dependence if he could in any way be forced to love, even if only to the slightest degree. Thus the "I" will be the pledge for the highest goal of man. But at the same time, if it does not discover love, if it hardens within itself, it is the tempter that plunges him into the abyss. For it is that which separates people from one another, which brings them to the great War of All against All, not only to the war of nation against nation.[40]

What protects us from falling into the abyss is our constant struggling for balance, for our point of equilibrium, our humanity, which we can glimpse in the Christ being. The experience of the middle, the central balancing realm is, at the same time, a conscious experience of the threshold, of the bridge between the world of matter and the world of the spirit.

---

[38] Rudolf Steiner: *Soziales Verständnis aus geisteswissenschaftlicher Erkenntnis*. Rudolf Steiner Verlag 1989 (vol. GA 191); Rudolf Steiner: *Atlantis and Lemuria*. Fredonia Books 2002 (vol. GA 11). The Bible speaks of Diabolos (Lucifer) and Satanas (Ahriman)

[39] Peter Selg: *Die "Wärme-Meditation": Geschichtlicher Hintergrund und ideelle Beziehungen*. Verlag am Goetheanum 2013

[40] Rudolf Steiner: *The Apocalypse of St. John*. Kessinger Publishing 2010 (vol. GA 104), lecture of 25 June 1908

The highest that can be given to us is the message of Christ Jesus. We must take it up thoroughly, not merely with our understanding; we must take it into our innermost being, just as one takes nourishment into the physical body.[41]

What unites us in the Anthroposophical Society since the Christmas Foundation Meeting is the great mutual task of helping to awaken in present day human beings a consciousness of the threshold to the spiritual world, so that increasing numbers of individual human beings can come to self-awareness and gain a connection to the great goals and tasks of humanity's evolution. This can only succeed, however, if as many people as possible can recognize and take seriously the social edifice that Rudolf Steiner was still able to found before his death – the Anthroposophical Society and the School of Spiritual Science with its various sections. This social framework offers opportunities for practice which can help us realize the impulse of the new Mysteries. For this impulse can take hold wherever community building succeeds in the light of the future ideals of humanity mentioned, when *many are united at the right time.*

Secrecy and Openness

The principle of secrecy, which had been a central aspect in the care of ancient Mystery knowledge, is subject to quite different conditions in the new Mysteries. Here one must respond to every seeker of knowledge, as Rudolf Steiner writes in his book of schooling, but one must also learn to remain silent when something is not asked.[42] The central element of the new Mysteries is rather what is done openly – as it should be for something of cultural value. It cannot be betrayed by any power in the world because it is not dependent upon a particular kind of knowledge that we have to have. What is crucial is solely what is achieved and therefore manifested. And if the good is done, then it reveals itself to the world, and has no need of secrecy.

The Key to the Raphael Mystery

But how can this new Mystery principle become fruitful for medical diagnostics and therapy? How can we take hold of the secret of the Mercury staff that brings the forces of "above and below" to the right place again?

---

[41] Ibid.

[42] Rudolf Steiner: *How to know Higher Worlds - A Modern Path of Initiation.* Anthroposophic Press 1994 (vol. GA 10), Chap. Initiation

Ita Wegman describes the key to this Raphael Mystery in her preface to the book *Fundamentals of Therapy* that Rudolf Steiner and she wrote together. Rudolf Steiner did not use her preface in the published book. It was preserved though and was published for the first time by Walter Holtzapfel, the leader of the Medical Section from 1969 to 1977, in a circular letter of the Section.[43]

Ita Wegman describes two main causes of illness seen from a physical and a spiritual point of view. *A sick person is always a completely individual case. There are no two people who can be sick in the same way. The things of nature which are not spiritual go back to general laws. What is individual is always an expression of the activity of soul-spiritual laws. These laws are not grasped in concepts but are only accessible to observation. (...)*

The soul-exercises that lead to spiritual perception consist either of a dampening or of an intensification of the life of soul. The dampening of the soul-life is an imitation of the illnesses of the first kind within the soul. The intensification of the soul-life is an imitation of the illnesses of the second kind. When we know the soul condition derived from such exercises, we also know the illnesses, for we have pictures of them in our soul conditions. If we describe the physical symptoms of illnesses by what we experience in these pictures, then we provide for every doctor descriptions that he can examine. If the description holds up to the investigation, the indications of spiritual research are confirmed. And if the doctor takes in the descriptions of such spiritual research again and again, then, through his portrayals of the complex of symptoms, he can gradually acquire the spiritual insights himself. We are of the opinion that the correct reading of this book will make it possible for every doctor to behold the illnesses himself spiritually.[44]

It is about the understanding that the path of practice from *How to know Higher Worlds* is connected with effort and soul-pains that are similar to those that the body suffers when it is ill. Illness appears to spiritual perception as a force-complex that should have been activated in the soul but now becomes engaged at the wrong place, in the body. The task of the physician, therefore, is to see behind every bodily illness the spiritual reality that is manifesting in this illness at the wrong place. With this we become aware of the meaning of illness in individual destiny, and we see

---

[43] Reprinted in: *Rundbrief für die Mitarbeiter der Medizinischen Sektion am Goetheanum in aller Welt.* Advent 1993, no. 2

[44] Ita Wegman: unpublished preface to the book *Fundamentals of Therapy.* See p. 41-43

illness as a *physical Imagination of spiritual life*,[45] as Rudolf Steiner formulates it in his *Course for Young Doctors* in 1924. In this context therapy means that the physical-imaginative aspect is on the road to recovery, to its proper place. Seen as such, the book of self-schooling by Rudolf Steiner, *How to Know Higher Worlds*, could also be read from the point of view of which illness can be prevented by working with a particular exercise described in the book.

The Example of Smallpox

In his *Course for Young Doctors* Rudolf Steiner describes smallpox as having its healthy spiritual counter-picture in a heavenly Imagination:

Think of the illness of smallpox which reveals itself in physical symptoms. But suppose you were able to do the following: picture to yourselves a person suffering from smallpox who in his astral body and ego organization had the power today to draw out the whole illness and to experience it only in the astral body and in the ego, so that in that moment his physical and ether bodies would be well. Suppose such a thing were hypothetically possible. What I have said cannot actually happen, but if you want to have this imagination you must do the same thing as I have described as a hypothetical case, without your physical body and ether body having smallpox. In the astral body and ego-organization, free from the physical and ether bodies, you must experience the illness of smallpox. In other words: you must experience, spiritually, a spiritual correlate of physical illness. The illness of smallpox is the physical image of the condition in which ego-organization and astral body are when they have such an imagination. You will realize now that in smallpox there is proceeding, but in this case from the human being himself, the same influence out of which, in spiritual knowledge, the heavenly imagination comes.

You see (...) how closely illness is related to the spiritual life – not to the physical body; illness is closely related to the spiritual life. Illness is the physical imagination of the spiritual life and because the physical imagination is in the wrong, because it ought not to imitate certain spiritual processes – therefore that which in the spiritual world may be something very sublime, is, under certain circumstances, illness in the physical organization.

---

[45] Rudolf Steiner: *Course for Young Doctors*. Mercury Press 1997 (vol. GA 316), p. 104

In trying to understand the nature of illness we must say to ourselves: were it not possible for certain spiritual beings to be brought down into a realm where they do not rightly belong, then these beings would not be present even in the spiritual world. The close relationship of true spiritual knowledge with illness is clear from this. When we have spiritual knowledge we have knowledge of illness. If one has a heavenly imagination such as that of which I spoke, one knows what smallpox is, because it is only the physical projection of what is experienced spiritually. And so it is, really, with all knowledge of illness. We can say: if heaven, or indeed hell, take too strong a hold of the human being, he becomes ill; if they only take hold of his soul or his spirit, he becomes wiser, or cleverer, or a seer.[46]

How can we bring together the described heavenly Imagination, in which the five winter constellations that have more of a cosmic feminine side and the seven summer constellations with more of a cosmic masculine element show themselves in harmonious collaboration – how do we bring this together with smallpox? Which exercises in *How to know Higher Worlds* would be appropriate to show that the forces that should be developed by the practice of an exercise now manifest in the wrong place, as a physical Imagination of spiritual life? In *Manifestations of Karma* Rudolf Steiner calls smallpox an organ of lovelessness.[47] When love cannot be socially activated and bring forth creative organs in the interaction of masculine and feminine qualities, then the tendency to become infected with smallpox is aided. We also violate one of the first duties and practices of the spirit-pupil, that in our dealings with other human beings we should not discriminate among status, name, and ethnicity, nor in relation to gender. The latter is especially precarious. The many daily injustices, innuendos, indignities and insults that occur with regard to the different approaches and dealings between men and women could certainly be seen in this context as one aspect of schooling that is not happening at the right place.

Smallpox is very "social", not only because of the mode of transmission but also because of the high rate of contagion spreading this illness to as many as possible. It is also the way the symptoms develop, with high temperature as a physical expression of warmth – which actually should

---

[46] Rudolf Steiner: *Course for Young Doctors*. Mercury Press 1997 (vol. GA 316), lecture of 8 Jan. 1924

[47] Rudolf Steiner: *Manifestations of Karma*. Rudolf Steiner Press 2011 (vol. GA 120), lecture of 26 May 1910

be the soul-spiritual warmth of compassion and understanding – connects itself with the forming of blisters on the surface of the skin, the mucus membrane, and on the surface also of inner organs. As if the boundaries wanted to open themselves physically because being open with one another on the soul-level, and in the sense of destiny, has not been successful. We meet here a disease that is not typically an individual disease but rather manifests as an epidemic, an answer, and is a compensation of destiny for a development towards a social awakening, which needs "healing of destiny" through illness.

Autoimmune Diseases
Can we not see this kind of illness as a bodily projection of the exercise of "observing oneself as a stranger"? If this is not practiced in accord with the person's learning disposition for this life, then the person chooses as compensation the path through illness in order to reach the desired goal.

Acquired Immune Deficiency HIV
In the case of HIV the spiritual counterpart that calls forth the symptoms would be selflessness. The HIV-infected person experiences how his biological immune-system that must naturally be egoistic, becomes more and more "altruistic", i.e. more selfless, and ever weaker. Thus the spiritual counterpart, the thing at the wrong place which calls forth the symptoms of the illness, is the quality of selflessness. Selfless service to all of humanity is t h e compensation for a materialistic world-conception and the presently prevailing cultural attitude. Selfless readiness to serve is the basis for the Christian-Rosicrucian path of schooling that Rudolf Steiner describes in his lectures on spiritual schooling: *The [spiritual pupil] does not learn in order to pile up treasures of knowledge, but rather to place what he has learned in the service of the world.*[48] HIV can therefore also be seen as a typical illness of our time. One part of humanity compensates for what has been caused by another. We see that many people have to suffer – especially in Africa – while the initiators of the materialistic conception can have the knowledge to protect themselves. However, in a following life those with this illness will be incarnating again with the fruits of the illness: a disposition toward selflessness and an inner strength.

---

[48] Rudolf Steiner: *How to know Higher Worlds - A Modern Path of Initiation.* Anthroposophic Press 1994 (vol. GA 10), Chap. Conditions

Oncological Illnesses

What spiritual aspect forms itself physically in the genesis of oncological disease patterns? How do they start? Some cell begins to be less specialized than it was. It moves out of its differentiation in an organ area back in the direction of its embryological origin, where it was hardly specialized and therefore more omnipotent. Normally, the immune system recognizes such cells and kills them. However, when the immune competence weakens or a disposition for a certain cancer has already made inroads, then the cancer begins to grow locally. It breaks through the basal membrane and begins to infiltrate and flourish. After that, metastasis occurs. Single cells separate off and begin to wander through the organism. Parallel to this, the overall health of the person changes. Cancer is a general disease. Appetite, awareness of life, sleeping/waking and the rhythms of the heart and breathing change. As a rule, the temperature curve becomes flat, sometimes even rigid, without morning and evening differences. If we let all of this work on us and inquire about such a disease process, then we see unpredictability. Bodily functions get out of control. Through metastasis, beginnings of new organs form somewhere indiscriminately. Order, control and the ability to integrate disappear and yield to arbitrariness, with its loss of differentiation, loss of restraint. What is it that projects itself in cancer as the "physical Imagination of spiritual life"? What signature, Imagination, characteristic does it represent? The signature of this course of illness is clear: cancer brings a "freedom impulse" to the physical-physiological level. Cancer is an illness where the freedom-impulse cannot manifest itself in the soul and spirit in the way that is needed for this person's destiny. This signature fits into our time, for we experience that the triumphal procession of this illness has until now been unstoppable. Every person now basically stands before the developmental task to realize his identity as a human being and use his freedom constructively.[49] Unconsciously the human being experiences in his course of illness what he actually wished to learn consciously. With this then, he develops the aptitude in a next life to develop freedom.

Rheumatism

Especially impressive in this respect is the example of rheumatism. Here we can see how the limb, immobilized by pain, displays in these bodily

---

[49] See also Michaela Glöckler: *Can Cancer Be Prevented?* Der Merkurstab 62:416-420, 2009

symptoms the first central exercise in Rudolf Steiner's book *How to know higher Worlds,* where we read: *Create for yourself moments of peace and learn at these moments to distinguish the essential from the non-essential.*[50] It occurs again and again that patients ask what they themselves can do for their recovery. In such cases it can be meaningful to name the counterpart of the illness and in case of a painful constriction of movement, recommend, for instance, this meditation:

> *I carry calm within me,*
> *I bear within myself*
> *The forces to make me strong.*
> *Now I will fill myself*
> *With their glowing warmth,*
> *Now I will imbue myself*
> *With my own will's resolve.*
> *And I will feel*
> *How calmness pours*
> *Through all my being,*
> *When I strengthen myself*
> *To find within myself*
> *Calmness as strength*
> *Through my striving's power.*[51]

When the ailing person does not ask, the doctor should not speak about the spiritual background of the disease process. The danger would otherwise exist that the described facts would awaken in the patient feelings of guilt that would intensify the symptoms of the disease. The doctor, however, should have this spiritual counter-part of the illness in his consciousness when he sees the patient. Then he works in a healing way on the patient just through his presence. In addition, this is for the doctor the best path for the prevention of disease. For when he lives in the counter-pictures of the diseases with his soul and spirit, by working with the exercises, loving them and living with them, then the possibility of their working in the wrong place disappears. In Anthroposophic Medicine we

---

[50] Rudolf Steiner: *How to know Higher Worlds - A Modern Path of Initiation.* Anthroposophic Press 1994 (vol. GA 10), Chap. The Preparation
[51] Rudolf Steiner: *Verses and Meditations.* Rudolf Steiner Press 2004 (vol. GA 268), p. 187

thus have in addition to the methods of conventional and alternative medicine the possibility of acquiring a deeper spiritual understanding of prevention, illness and healing in their interrelatedness. Learning to work with these insights therapeutically can contribute to the nature and content of a Raphael school.

Ita Wegman's Preface to the Book
Fundamentals of Therapy[52]

In our time, medicine has taken on a purely scientific character. With this it became totally dependent on the views that developed in the present time concerning science and scientific methods. According to these views we only accept as scientific what can be determined by sense perceptible observation, through experimentation or by rational deduction from these. We must ask ourselves: Are the scientific results gained in this way applicable to the individual human being? We may have noticed common human characteristics in so and so many human beings, however, the individual being of a single person is only understandable when we have the gift of direct observation of what is individual. A sick person is always a completely individual case. There are no two people that can be sick in the same way. The things of nature that are not spiritual go back to general laws. What is individual is always an expression of the activity of soul-spiritual laws. These laws are not grasped in concepts but are only accessible to observation. We will speak in this book of a medical system that is built on the observation of the spirit, in the same way that natural law is built on the sense-world. We know that many will believe us to be in opposition to the recognized natural-scientific direction of medicine. This will most certainly not be the case. We fully acknowledge today's results of this direction. It is undeniable though, that this direction of medicine must come to a halt before the true nature of illness. It can speak about the harm to the organism and its members, but it cannot gain insight into why an organism would develop harmful effects out of itself. The natural scientific direction of the organism lies in its development from seed to full maturity. Within this development, stopping short at what is natural, we will not find the forces that can obstruct this development. In illness, though, these forces are at work.

Where do they come from?
We will only be able to answer this question when we look at the – in a certain way – exaggerated natural evolution of the human being. Everywhere where such an exaggeration happens, unconscious activity takes

---

[52] This manuscript in Ita Wegman's handwriting was discovered among her things in the early 1970s and initially published in the Newsletter of the Medical Section at the Goetheanum (no. 6, 1 May 1973). It is a concept by Ita Wegman, whose content reappears in the first and second chapters of *Fundamentals of Therapy*.

over and consciousness retreats. From this we can conclude that the forces underlying consciousness, the spiritual forces, work in the opposite direction from the natural. This means that they must be catabolic forces, while the natural forces are anabolic. A human in a certain condition of health, and with a normal consciousness has within him a certain state of balance between the anabolic and catabolic forces. When this balance is disturbed then there is illness. This can happen in two ways. The anabolic forces can become too strong, then they weaken the spiritual forces. This is one form of illness. It happens, when for instance, the regenerating metabolic processes in the brain are too strong. Then consciousness is dampened.

The other form of illness occurs when the catabolic forces become too strong. Then an exaggerated working of consciousness occurs. We meet the other form of illness when forces work in the digestive system that should only work with such strength in the brain. The exaggerated working of consciousness manifests as pain, for pain is nothing other than a heightened condition of consciousness.

Illnesses of the first type can only occur in the organism when, underlying a normal condition, a strong catabolic activity is at work. If this is dampened down or lessened in its strength, then illness occurs.

Illnesses of the second kind can only happen when, underlying a normal condition, a strong anabolic, regenerative activity occurs. Dampening this activity means illness.

The first case is present in the human organism in all the organs that serve perception or thinking. A spiritual viewpoint makes immediately clear that perception and thinking are of a purely spiritual origin. A merely natural activity cannot be equated with perception and thinking. Rather, when perception and thinking should arise in the organism, the natural activity must lessen in order to make room for the spiritual. When, on the other hand natural activity is present in its full regenerating capacity, no spiritual activity can penetrate. This is the case with the metabolic system and with occurrences that underlie the movement of the organism. We can see here that as soon as we begin to observe an illness, we should keep an eye on the relationship of the natural and the spiritual activities.

Now, we have today a relatively complete science of the natural, but there is distance kept from a science of the spirit. In this book we will proceed from a science of the spirit in the same way as from a science of the natural. This presupposes that an observation of the spirit is acknowledged. This is not given to humans from the outset as is the case with the observation of the natural. We learn to perceive with our senses and we learn to use our conceptual power through our natural development and through our education. Spiritual observation has first to be gained. In this book illnesses and the healing process will be described as they are discovered by spiritual observation. This spiritual observation can be acquired through certain specific soul exercises. It will be objected that we cannot demand that every doctor do such exercises. An obvious objection against this book will therefore be: Its indications and statements cannot be examined by people who have not acquired a spiritual conception through such exercises.

We want to refute such objections. The soul-exercises that lead to spiritual perception consist either of a dampening or of an intensification of the soul-life. The dampening of the soul-life is within the soul an imitation of the illnesses of the first kind, an intensification of the soul-life is an imitation of the illnesses of the second kind. When we know the soul-condition that comes from such exercises, we also know the illnesses, for in the soul-conditions we have the pictures of them. If we describe the physical symptoms of illnesses by what we experience in these pictures, then we provide for every doctor the descriptions that he can examine. If the descriptions hold up to investigation, the indications of spiritual research are confirmed. And if the doctor takes in the descriptions of such spiritual research again and again, then, through his portrayals of the complex of symptoms, he can gradually acquire the spiritual insights himself. We are of the opinion that the correct reading of this book will make it possible for every doctor to behold the illnesses himself spiritually. However, we also know, since we believe that we understand human beings, that such reading will not take place in all cases because the readers will be annoyed by what they perceive as strange explanations. And between the spirit of some readers and the spirit of our book will be the anger of those that cannot get over the fact that we have to say something different from what they have said up to now.

Rudolf Steiner's Rose Cross Meditation[53]

One example of meditation based upon a symbolical concept will now be placed before the reader. Such a concept must first be built up in the soul, and this may be done in the following manner. Let us think of a plant, calling to mind how it is rooted in the ground, the way in which leaf after leaf shoots forth, until finally the blossom unfolds. And then let us imagine a human being placed beside this plant, and let us call up in our soul the thought that he has qualities and characteristics which, when compared with those of the plant, will be found to be more perfect. We dwell on the fact that this being is able to move here and there, according to his will and his desires, while the plant remains stationary, rooted in the soil.

But now let us also consider: Yes, man is certainly more perfect than the plant; but on the other hand, I find in him qualities which I cannot perceive in the plant and through the lack of which the plant appears more perfect than man in certain respects. Man is filled with passions and desires and these govern his conduct. With him we can speak of sin committed by reason of his impulses and passions, whereas in the plant, we see that it follows the pure laws of growth from leaf to leaf, and that the blossom without passion opens to the chaste rays of the sun. So we can see that man possesses a certain perfection beyond the plant, but that on the other hand he has paid for this perfection by admitting into his being inclinations, desires and passions in addition to the pure forces of the plant. And then we call to mind the green sap flowing through the plant, and think of it as the expression of the pure and passionless laws of growth. And then again, we call to mind the red blood as it courses through the veins of man, and we recognize in it an expression of man's instincts, his passions and desires. Let a vivid picture of all this arise in our souls. We then think of man's faculties of development; how he can purify and cleanse his inclinations and passions through his higher soul faculties. We think how through this process something that is low is destroyed in these inclinations and passions which thereby are born upon a higher plane. Then we may be able to think of the blood as the expression of these purified and cleansed inclinations and passions.

Now we gaze in spirit on the rose and say to ourselves: "In the red sap of the rose is the erstwhile green sap of the plant – now changed to crimson – and the red rose follows the same pure, passionless laws of growth as does the green leaf." Thus the red of the rose may offer us a symbol of

---

[53] Rudolf Steiner: *Occult Science.* Anthroposophic Press 2009 (vol. GA 13)

a kind of blood which is the expression of cleansed impulses and passions, purged of all lower elements, and resembling in their purity the forces working in the red rose. Let us now try not only to assimilate such thoughts within our reason, but also let them come to life within our feelings. We can experience a blissful sensation when contemplating the purity and passionless nature of the growing plant. We can awaken the feeling within us how certain higher perfections must be paid for through the acquisition of passions and desires. This, then, can change the blissful sensation previously experienced into a serious mood: and then only can it stir within us the feeling of liberating happiness, if we abandon ourselves to the thought of the red blood that can become the carrier of inner pure experiences, like the red sap of the rose.

The important point is that we should not look coldly and without feeling upon these thoughts which serve to build up such a symbolical concept. After dwelling for a time upon the above mentioned thoughts and feelings, let us try to transmute them into the following symbolical concept. Let us imagine a black cross. Let this be the symbol for the destroyed lower element of our desires and passions and there where the beams of the cross intersect, let us imagine seven red radiating roses arranged in a circle. Let these roses be the symbol for a blood that is the expression of cleansed and purified passions and desires.

Now we must call up this symbolical concept before our soul just as has been described in the case of a memory-concept. Such a concept has an awakening power if one abandons oneself to it in inner meditation. One must try during this meditation to exclude all other concepts. Only the described symbol must float before the soul as vividly as possible.

It is not without significance that this symbol has been introduced, not merely as an awakening percept, but because it has been constructed out of certain perceptions concerning plants and man. For the effect of such a symbol depends upon the fact of its being put together in this definite manner, before employing it as an instrument for meditation. Should it be called up without a previous process of construction such as has here been delineated, the picture must remain cold and will be far less effective than if it had by previous preparation gathered force with which to give warmth to the soul. During meditation, however, one should not call up in the soul all the preparatory thoughts, but merely allow the life-like image to float before one's mind and at the same time permit those feelings which are the result of these preparatory thoughts to vibrate with it. Thus the symbol becomes a sign, co-existent with the inner experience. And it is the dwelling of the soul in this experience that is the active principle.

The longer one can do this, without admitting disturbing impressions, the more effective will be the whole process.

It is well, however, in addition to the time used in meditation itself, to repeat the building up of the image through the feelings, as described above, so that the corresponding sensation may not pale. The greater the patience brought to bear in performing these acts of repetition, the more effective becomes this image for the soul.

The Mystery of the Mercury Staff: the Metamorphosis of Growth Forces into Thinking Forces

These forces functioning in the ether body are active at the beginning of the human being's life on earth – most distinctly during the embryonic period – as the forces of formation and growth. During the course of earthly life a portion of these forces emancipates itself from this occupation with formation and growth and becomes forces of thinking, just those forces which for the ordinary consciousness bring forth the shadowlike world of thoughts.

It is of the utmost importance to know that the human being's ordinary forces of thinking are refined formative and growth forces. A spiritual element reveals itself in the forming and growing of the human organism. And this spiritual element then appears during the course of later life as the spiritual power of thought.

This power of thought is only one part of the human capacity for form and growth that weaves in the etheric. The other part remains true to the purpose that it fulfilled in the beginning of the human being's life. Only because the human being continues to evolve even when his form and his growth are advanced, that is, when they are to a certain degree completed, does the etheric spiritual force, which lives and works in the organism, appear in later life as the power of thought.

To imaginative spiritual vision the sculpting force of one aspect thus reveals itself as an etheric spiritual element, and from another aspect it appears as the soul content of our thinking.[54]

Rudolf Steiner describes how, corresponding to the metamorphosis of growth forces into thinking forces, the astral body and "I"-organization "metamorphose" out of the physical body into thought forces during the course of growth and development, becoming free for the soul activities of feeling and willing. They do this "on the channels of the etheric". Where can this emancipation take place? There is only one organ in which the streaming blood as the carrier of the four ethers comes to a standstill and gives the possibility "to die", that is, to go out of the physical context: the heart. At the end of the diastole, in the "diastasis", there is a brief moment in which every bit of the streaming blood comes to a complete standstill, before the expelling phase of the systole begins. Our conscious soul life is as if born out of the foundations of the heart,[55,56] reflected in the brain and then used more or less freely, consciously and "cordially". "Thinking with the heart" has this special physiological connection. It happens when thoughts are "taken to heart" and continue to have an effect from there.

The collaboration of the two archangels Michael and Raphael is reflected in the physiological interaction between the heart (Michael) and lungs (Raphael). In the Parsifal legend they are represented by Parsifal (heart) and Gawan (lungs). Parsifal, who seeks a path through error and trials, and Gawan, who succeeds at everything and can bring healing and deliverance everywhere. These are the archetypes of self-healing (Parsifal) and therapy (Gawan).

---

[54] Rudolf Steiner, Ita Wegman: *Fundamentals of Therapy,* Mercury Press 1999, vol. GA 27, p. 11-12

[55] Michaela Glöckler (ed.): *Meditations on Heart-Activity by Rudolf Steiner.* Medical Section at the Goetheanum 2014

[56] Christoph Rubens, Peter Selg (ed.): *Das menschliche Herz. Kardiologie in der Anthroposophischen Medizin.* Ita Wegman Institut 2014

The Book of Tobit

1 The Piety, Misfortune and Prayer of the Elder Tobit

1 The book of the words of Tobit, son of Tobiel, the son of Ananiel, the son of Aduel, the son of Gabael, of the seed of Asael, of the tribe of Nephthali; 2 Who in the time of Enemessar king of the Assyrians was led captive out of Thisbe, which is at the right hand of that city, which is called properly Nephthali in Galilee above Aser. 3 I Tobit have walked all the days of my life in the ways of truth and justice, and I did many almsdeeds to my brethren, and my nation, who came with me to Nineve, into the land of the Assyrians.

4 And when I was in mine own country, in the land of Israel being but young, all the tribe of Nephthali my father fell from the house of Jerusalem, which was chosen out of all the tribes of Israel, that all the tribes should sacrifice there, where the temple of the habitation of the most High was consecrated and built for all ages. 5 Now all the tribes which together revolted, and the house of my father Nephthali, sacrificed unto the heifer Baal. 6 But I alone went often to Jerusalem at the feasts, as it was ordained unto all the people of Israel by an everlasting decree, having the first fruits and tenths of increase, with that which was first shorn; and them gave I at the altar to the priests the children of Aaron. 7 The first tenth part of all increase I gave to the sons of Aaron, who ministered at Jerusalem: another tenth part I sold away, and went, and spent it every year at Jerusalem: 8 And the third I gave unto them to whom it was meet, as Debora my father's mother had commanded me, because I was left an orphan by my father. 9 Furthermore, when I was come to the age of a man, I married Anna of mine own kindred, and of her I begat Tobias. 10 And when we were carried away captives to Nineve, all my brethren and those that were of my kindred did eat of the bread of the Gentiles.

11 But I kept myself from eating; 12 Because I remembered God with all my heart. 13 And the most High gave me grace and favour before Enemessar, so that I was his purveyor. 14 And I went into Media, and left in trust with Gabael, the brother of Gabrias, at Rages a city of Media ten talents of silver. 15 Now when Enemessar was dead, Sennacherib his son reigned in his stead; whose estate was troubled, that I could not go into Media. 16 And in the time of Enemessar I gave many alms to my brethren, and gave my bread to the hungry, 17 And my clothes to the naked: and if I saw any of my nation dead, or cast about the walls of Nineve, I buried him.

18 And if the king Sennacherib had slain any, when he was come, and fled from Judea, I buried them privily; for in his wrath he killed many; but the bodies were not found, when they were sought for of the king. **19** And when one of the Ninevites went and complained of me to the king, that I buried them, and hid myself; understanding that I was sought for to be put to death, I withdrew myself for fear. **20** Then all my goods were forcibly taken away, neither was there any thing left me, beside my wife Anna and my son Tobias.

21 And there passed not five and fifty days, before two of his sons killed him, and they fled into the mountains of Ararath; and Sarchedonus his son reigned in his stead; who appointed over his father's accounts, and over all his affairs, Achiacharus my brother Anael's son. **22** And Achiacharus intreating for me, I returned to Nineve. Now Achiacharus was cupbearer, and keeper of the signet, and steward, and overseer of the accounts: and Sarchedonus appointed him next unto him: and he was my brother's son.

2

1 Now when I was come home again, and my wife Anna was restored unto me, with my son Tobias, in the feast of Pentecost, which is the holy feast of the seven weeks, there was a good dinner prepared me, in the which I sat down to eat. **2** And when I saw abundance of meat, I said to my son, Go and bring what poor man soever thou shalt find out of our brethren, who is mindful of the Lord; and, lo, I tarry for thee. **3** But he came again, and said, Father, one of our nation is strangled, and is cast out in the marketplace. **4** Then before I had tasted of any meat, I started up, and took him up into a room until the going down of the sun. **5** Then I returned, and washed myself, and ate my meat in heaviness, **6** Remembering that prophecy of Amos, as he said, Your feasts shall be turned into mourning, and all your mirth into lamentation. **7** Therefore I wept: and after the going down of the sun I went and made a grave, and buried him.

8 But my neighbours mocked me, and said, This man is not yet afraid to be put to death for this matter: who fled away; and yet, lo, he burieth the dead again. **9** The same night also I returned from the burial, and slept by the wall of my courtyard, being polluted and my face was uncovered:

10 And I knew not that there were sparrows in the wall, and mine eyes being open, the sparrows muted warm dung into mine eyes, and a whiteness came in mine eyes: and I went to the physicians, but they helped me not: moreover Achiacharus did nourish me, until I went into Elymais. **11** And my wife Anna did take women's works to do. **12** And when she had sent them home to the owners, they paid her wages, and gave her also besides a kid. **13** And when it was in my house, and began to cry, I said unto her, From whence is this kid? is it not stolen? render it to the owners; for it is not lawful to eat any thing that is stolen. **14** But she replied upon me, It was given for a gift more than the wages. Howbeit I did not believe her, but bade her render it to the owners: and I was abashed at her. But she replied upon me, Where are thine alms and thy righteous deeds? behold, thou and all thy works are known.

3

1 Then I being grieved did weep, and in my sorrow prayed, saying, **2** O Lord, thou art just, and all thy works and all thy ways are mercy and truth, and thou judgest truly and justly for ever. **3** Remember me, and look on me, punish me not for my sins and ignorances, and the sins of my fathers, who have sinned before thee: **4** For they obeyed not thy commandments: wherefore thou hast delivered us for a spoil, and unto captivity, and unto death, and for a proverb of reproach to all the nations among whom we are dispersed. **5** And now thy judgments are many and true: deal with me according to my sins and my fathers': because we have not kept thy commandments, neither have walked in truth before thee. **6** Now therefore deal with me as seemeth best unto thee, and command my spirit to be taken from me, that I may be dissolved, and become earth: for it is profitable for me to die rather than to live, because I have heard false reproaches, and have much sorrow: command therefore that I may now be delivered out of this distress, and go into the everlasting place: turn not thy face away from me.

Sara's Troubles and Prayer

7 It came to pass the same day, that in Ecbatane a city of Media Sara the daughter of Raguel was also reproached by her father's maids; **8** Because that she had been married to seven husbands, whom Asmodeus the evil spirit had killed, before they had lain with her. Dost thou not know, said they, that thou hast strangled thine husbands? thou hast had already seven husbands, neither wast thou named after any of them. **9** Wherefore dost thou beat us for them? if they be dead, go thy ways after them, let us never see of thee either son or daughter. **10** Whe she heard these things, she was very sorrowful, so that she thought to have strangled herself; and she said, I am the only daughter of my father, and if I do this, it shall be a reproach unto him, and I shall bring his old age with sorrow unto the grave. **11** Then she prayed toward the window, and said, Blessed art thou, O Lord my God, and thine holy and glorious name is blessed and honourable for ever: let all thy works praise thee for ever. **12** And now, O Lord, I set mine eyes and my face toward thee,

13 And say, Take me out of the earth, that I may hear no more the reproach. **14** Thou knowest, Lord, that I am pure from all sin with man, **15** And that I never polluted my name, nor the name of my father, in the land of my captivity: I am the only daughter of my father, neither hath he any child to be his heir, neither any near kinsman, nor any son of his alive, to whom I may keep myself for a wife: my seven husbands are already dead; and why should I live? but if it please not thee that I should die, command some regard to be had of me, and pity taken of me, that I hear no more reproach.

The answer to her prayers

16 So the prayers of them both were heard before the majesty of the great God. **17** And Raphael was sent to heal them both, that is, to scale away the whiteness of Tobit's eyes, and to give Sara the daughter of Raguel for a wife to Tobias the son of Tobit; and to bind Asmodeus the evil spirit; because she belonged to Tobias by right of inheritance. The selfsame time came Tobit home, and entered into his house, and Sara the daughter of Raguel came down from her upper chamber.

4 Tobit's legacy

1 In that day Tobit remembered the money which he had committed to Gabael in Rages of Media, **2** And said with himself, I have wished for death; wherefore do I not call for my son Tobias that I may signify to him of the money before I die? **3** And when he had called him, he said, My son, when I am dead, bury me; and despise not thy mother, but honour her all the days of thy life, and do that which shall please her, and grieve her not. **4** Remember, my son, that she saw many dangers for thee, when thou wast in her womb: and when she is dead, bury her by me in one grave.

5 My son, be mindful of the Lord our God all thy days, and let not thy will be set to sin, or to transgress his commandments: do uprightly all thy life long, and follow not the ways of unrighteousness. **6** For if thou deal truly, thy doings shall prosperously succeed to thee, and to all them that live justly. **7** Give alms of thy substance; and when thou givest alms, let not thine eye be envious, neither turn thy face from any poor, and the face of God shall not be turned away from thee. **8** If thou hast abundance give alms accordingly: if thou have but a little, be not afraid to give according to that little: **9** For thou layest up a good treasure for thyself against the day of necessity. **10** Because that alms do deliver from death, and suffereth not to come into darkness. **11** For alms is a good gift unto all that give it in the sight of the most High.

12 Beware of all whoredom, my son, and chiefly take a wife of the seed of thy fathers, and take not a strange woman to wife, which is not of thy father's tribe: for we are the children of the prophets, Noe, Abraham, Isaac, and Jacob: remember, my son, that our fathers from the beginning, even that they all married wives of their own kindred, and were blessed in their children, and their seed shall inherit the land. **13** Now therefore, my son, love thy brethren, and despise not in thy heart thy brethren, the sons and daughters of thy people, in not taking a wife of them: for in pride is destruction and much trouble, and in lewdness is decay and great want: for lewdness is the mother of famine. **14** Let not the wages of any man, which hath wrought for thee, tarry with thee, but give him it out of hand: for if thou serve God, he will also repay thee: be circumspect my son, in all things thou doest, and be wise in all thy conversation. **15** Do that to no man which thou hatest: drink not wine to make thee drunken: neither let drunkenness go with thee in thy journey. **16** Give of thy bread to the hungry, and of thy garments to them that are naked; and according to thine abundance give alms: and let not thine eye be envious, when thou givest alms. **17** Pour out thy bread on the burial of the just, but give nothing to the wicked. **18** Ask counsel of all that are wise, and despise not any counsel that is profitable. **19** Bless the Lord thy God alway, and desire of him that thy ways may be directed, and that all thy paths and counsels may prosper: for every nation hath not counsel; but the Lord himself giveth all good things, and he humbleth whom he will, as he will; now therefore, my son, remember my commandments, neither let them be put out of thy mind.

20 And now I signify this to they that I committed ten talents to Gabael the son of Gabrias at Rages in Media. **21** And fear not, my son, that we are made poor: for thou hast much wealth, if thou fear God, and depart from all sin, and do that which is pleasing in his sight.

5 The companion of Tobias the younger
1 Tobias then answered and said, Father, I will do all things which thou hast commanded me: **2** But how can I receive the money, seeing I know him not? **3** Then he gave him the handwriting, and said unto him, Seek thee a man which may go with thee, whiles I yet live, and I will give him wages: and go and receive the money.

4 Therefore when he went to seek a man, he found Raphael that was an angel. **5** But he knew not; and he said unto him, Canst thou go with me to Rages? and knowest thou those places well? **6** To whom the angel said, I will go with thee, and I know the way well: for I have lodged with our brother Gabael. **7** Then Tobias said unto him, Tarry for me, till I tell my father.

The companion of Tobit the younger
8 Then he said unto him, Go and tarry not. So he went in and said to his father, Behold, I have found one which will go with me. Then he said, Call him unto me, that I may know of what tribe he is, and whether he be a trusty man to go with thee. **9** So he called him, and he came in, and they saluted one another. **10** Then Tobit said unto him, Brother, shew me of what tribe and family thou art. **11** To whom he said, Dost thou seek for a tribe or family, or an hired man to go with thy son? Then Tobit said unto him, I would know, brother, thy kindred and name. **12** Then he said, I am Azarias, the son of Ananias the great, and of thy brethren. **13** Then Tobit said, Thou art welcome, brother; be not now angry with me, because I have enquired to know thy tribe and thy family; for thou art my brother, of an honest and good stock: for I know Ananias and Jonathas, sons of that great Samaias, as we went together to Jerusalem to worship, and offered the firstborn, and the tenths of the fruits; and they were not seduced with the error of our brethren: my brother, thou art of a good stock. **14** But tell me, what wages shall I give thee? wilt thou a drachm a day, and things necessary, as to mine own son? **15** Yea, moreover, if ye return safe, I will add something to thy wages.

Saying farewell to his parents
16 So they were well pleased. Then said he to Tobias, Prepare thyself for the journey, and God send you a good journey. And when his son had prepared all things for the journey, his father said, Go thou with this man, and God, which dwelleth in heaven, prosper your journey, and the angel of God keep you company. So they went forth both, and the young man's dog with them. **17** But Anna his mother wept, and said to Tobit, Why hast thou sent away our son? is he not the staff of our hand, in going in and out before us? **18** Be not greedy to add money to money: but let it be as refuse in respect of our child. **19** For that which the Lord hath given us to live with doth suffice us. **20** Then said Tobit to her, Take no care, my sister; he shall return in safety, and thine eyes shall see him. **21** For the

good angel will keep him company, and his journey shall be prosperous, and he shall return safe. **22** Then she made an end of weeping.

6 The large fish and the Angel's advice

1 And as they went on their journey, they came in the evening to the river Tigris, and they lodged there. **2** And when the young man went down to wash himself, a fish leaped out of the river, and would have devoured him.

3 Then the angel said unto him, Take the fish. And the young man laid hold of the fish, and drew it to land. **4** To whom the angel said, Open the fish, and take the heart and the liver and the gall, and put them up safely. **5** So the young man did as the angel commanded him; and when they had roasted the fish, they did eat it: then they both went on their way, till they drew near to Ecbatane. **6** Then the young man said to the angel, Brother Azarias, to what use is the heart and the liver and the gal of the fish? **7** And he said unto him, Touching the heart and the liver, if a devil or an evil spirit trouble any, we must make a smoke thereof before the man or the woman, and the party shall be no more vexed. **8** As for the gall, it is good to anoint a man that hath whiteness in his eyes, and he shall be healed. **9** And when they were come near to Rages,

10 The angel said to the young man, Brother, to day we shall lodge with Raguel, who is thy cousin; he also hath one only daughter, named Sara; I will speak for her, that she may be given thee for a wife. **11** For to thee doth the right of her appertain, seeing thou only art of her kindred. **12** And the maid is fair and wise: now therefore hear me, and I will speak to her father; and when we return from Rages we will celebrate the marriage: for I know that Raguel cannot marry her to another according to the law of Moses, but he shall be guilty of death, because the right of inheritance doth rather appertain to thee than to any other. **13** Then the young man answered the angel, I have heard, brother Azarias that this maid hath been given to seven men, who all died in the marriage chamber. **14** And now I am the only son of my father, and I am afraid, lest if I go in unto her, I die, as the other before: for a wicked spirit loveth her, which hurteth no body, but those which come unto her; wherefore I also fear lest I die, and bring my father's and my mother's life because of me to the grave with sorrow: for they have no other son to bury them.

15 Then the angel said unto him, Dost thou not remember the precepts which thy father gave thee, that thou shouldest marry a wife of thine own kindred? wherefore hear me, O my brother; for she shall be given thee to wife; and make thou no reckoning of the evil spirit; for this same night shall she be given thee in marriage. **16** And when thou shalt come into the marriage chamber, thou shalt take the ashes of perfume, and shalt lay upon them some of the heart and liver of the fish, and shalt make a smoke with it: **17** And the devil shall smell it, and flee away, and never come again any more: but when thou shalt come to her, rise up both of you, and pray to God which is merciful, who will have pity on you, and save you: fear not, for she is appointed unto thee from the beginning; and thou shalt preserve her, and she shall go with thee. Moreover I suppose that she shall bear thee children. Now when Tobias had heard these things, he loved her, and his heart was effectually joined to her.

7 Tobias marries Sara

1 And when they were come to Ecbatane, they came to the house of Raguel, and Sara met them: and after they had saluted one another, she brought them into the house. **2** Then said Raguel to Edna his wife, How like is this young man to Tobit my cousin! **3** And Raguel asked them, From whence are ye, brethren? To whom they said, We are of the sons of Nephthalim, which are captives in Nineve. **4** Then he said to them, Do ye know Tobit our kinsman? And they said, We know him. Then said he, Is he in good health?

5 And they said, He is both alive, and in good health: and Tobias said, He is my father. **6** Then Raguel leaped up, and kissed him, and wept, **7** And blessed him, and said unto him, Thou art the son of an honest and good man. But when he had heard that Tobit was blind, he was sorrowful, and wept. **8** And likewise Edna his wife and Sara his daughter wept. Moreover they entertained them cheerfully; and after that they had killed a ram of the flock, they set store of meat on the table. Then said Tobias to Raphael, Brother Azarias, speak of those things of which thou didst talk in the way, and let this business be dispatched.

9 So he communicated the matter with Raguel: and Raguel said to Tobias, Eat and drink, and make merry: **10** For it is meet that thou shouldest marry my daughter: nevertheless I will declare unto thee the truth. **11** I have given my daughter in marriage to seven men, who died that night they came in unto her: nevertheless for the present be merry. But Tobias said, I will eat nothing here, till we agree and swear one to another. **12** Raguel said, Then take her from henceforth according to the manner, for thou art her cousin, and she is thine, and the merciful God give you good success in all things. **13** Then he called his daughter Sara, and she came to her father, and he took her by the hand, and gave her to be wife to Tobias, saying, Behold, take her after the law of Moses, and lead her away to thy father. And he blessed them; **14** And called Edna his wife, and took paper, and did write an instrument of covenants, and sealed it. **15** Then they began to eat.

16 After Raguel called his wife Edna, and said unto her, Sister, prepare another chamber, and bring her in thither. **17** Which when she had done as he had bidden her, she brought her thither: and she wept, and she received the tears of her daughter, and said unto her, **18** Be of good comfort, my daughter; the Lord of heaven and earth give thee joy for this thy sorrow: be of good comfort, my daughter.

8 Wedding night and feast

1 And when they had supped, they brought Tobias in unto her. **2** And as he went, he remembered the words of Raphael, and took the ashes of the perfumes, and put the heart and the liver of the fish thereupon, and made a smoke therewith. **3** The which smell when the evil spirit had smelled, he fled into the utmost parts of Egypt, and the angel bound him.

4 And after that they were both shut in together, Tobias rose out of the bed, and said, Sister, arise, and let us pray that God would have pity on us. **5** Then began Tobias to say, Blessed art thou, O God of our fathers, and blessed is thy holy and glorious name for ever; let the heavens bless thee, and all thy creatures. **6** Thou madest Adam, and gavest him Eve his wife for an helper and stay: of them came mankind: thou hast said, It is not good that man should be alone; let us make unto him an aid like unto himself.

7 And now, O Lord, I take not this my sister for lust but uprightly: therefore mercifully ordain that we may become aged together. **8** And she said with him, Amen. **9** So they slept both that night. And Raguel arose, and went and made a grave, **10** Saying, I fear lest he also be dead. **11** But when Raguel was come into his house,

12 He said unto his wife Edna. Send one of the maids, and let her see whether he be alive: if he be not, that we may bury him, and no man know it. **13** So the maid opened the door, and went in, and found them both asleep, **14** And came forth, and told them that he was alive.

15 Then Raguel praised God, and said, O God, thou art worthy to be praised with all pure and holy praise; therefore let thy saints praise thee with all thy creatures; and let all thine angels and thine elect praise thee for ever. **16** Thou art to be praised, for thou hast made me joyful; and that is not come to me which I suspected; but thou hast dealt with us according to thy great mercy. **17** Thou art to be praised because thou hast had mercy of two that were the only begotten children of their fathers: grant them mercy, O Lord, and finish their life in health with joy and mercy. **18** Then Raguel bade his servants to fill the grave.

19 And he kept the wedding feast fourteen days. **20** For before the days of the marriage were finished, Raguel had said unto him by an oath, that he should not depart till the fourteen days of the marriage were expired; **21** And then he should take the half of his goods, and go in safety to his father; and should have the rest when I and my wife be dead.

9 Gabael at the wedding

1 Then Tobias called Raphael, and said unto him, **2** Brother Azarias, take with thee a servant, and two camels, and go to Rages of Media to Gabael, and bring me the money, and bring him to the wedding. **3** For Raguel hath sworn that I shall not depart. **4** But my father counteth the days; and if I tarry long, he will be very sorry. **5** So Raphael went out, and lodged with Gabael, and gave him the handwriting: who brought forth bags which were sealed up, and gave them to him. **6** And early in the morning they went forth both together, and came to the wedding: and Tobias blessed his wife.

10 The parents worry about their son

1 Now Tobit his father counted every day: and when the days of the journey were expired, and they came not, **2** Then Tobit said, Are they detained? or is Gabael dead, and there is no man to give him the money? **3** Therefore he was very sorry. **4** Then his wife said unto him, My son is dead, seeing he stayeth long; and she began to wail him, and said, **5** Now I care for nothing, my son, since I have let thee go, the light of mine eyes.

6 To whom Tobit said, Hold thy peace, take no care, for he is safe. **7** But she said, Hold thy peace, and deceive me not; my son is dead. And she went out every day into the way which they went, and did eat no meat on the daytime, and ceased not whole nights to bewail her son Tobias, until the fourteen days of the wedding were expired, which Raguel had sworn that he should spend there. Then Tobias said to Raguel, Let me go, for my father and my mother look no more to see me. **8** But his father in law said unto him, Tarry with me, and I will send to thy father, and they shall declare unto him how things go with thee. **9** But Tobias said, No; but let me go to my father.

10 Then Raguel arose, and gave him Sara his wife, and half his goods, servants, and cattle, and money: **11** And he blessed them, and sent them away, saying, The God of heaven give you a prosperous journey, my children. **12** And he said to his daughter, Honour thy father and thy mother in law, which are now thy parents, that I may hear good report of thee. And he kissed her. Edna also said to Tobias, The Lord of heaven restore thee, my dear brother, and grant that I may see thy children of my daughter Sara before I die, that I may rejoice before the Lord: behold, I commit my daughter unto thee of special trust; where are do not entreat her evil.

11 Homecoming and healing

1 After these things Tobias went his way, praising God that he had given him a prosperous journey, and blessed Raguel and Edna his wife, and went on his way till they drew near unto Nineve. 2 Then Raphael said to Tobias, Thou knowest, brother, how thou didst leave thy father: 3 Let us haste before thy wife, and prepare the house. 4 And take in thine hand the gall of the fish. So they went their way, and the dog went after them.

5 Now Anna sat looking about toward the way for her son. 6 And when she espied him coming, she said to his father, Behold, thy son cometh, and the man that went with him.

7 Then said Raphael, I know, Tobias, that thy father will open his eyes. 8 Therefore anoint thou his eyes with the gall, and being pricked therewith, he shall rub, and the whiteness shall fall away, and he shall see thee. 9 Then Anna ran forth, and fell upon the neck of her son, and said unto him, Seeing I have seen thee, my son, from henceforth I am content to die. And they wept both. 10 Tobit also went forth toward the door, and stumbled: but his son ran unto him, 11 And took hold of his father: and he strake of the gall on his father's eyes, saying, Be of good hope, my father. 12 And when his eyes began to smart, he rubbed them; 13 And the whiteness pilled away from the corners of his eyes: and when he saw his son, he fell upon his neck.

14 And he wept, and said, Blessed art thou, O God, and blessed is thy name for ever; and blessed are all thine holy angels: 15 For thou hast scourged, and hast taken pity on me: for, behold, I see my son Tobias. And his son went in rejoicing, and told his father the great things that had happened to him in Media. 16 Then Tobit went out to meet his daughter in law at the gate of Nineve, rejoicing and praising God: and they which saw him go marvelled, because he had received his sight.

17 But Tobias gave thanks before them, because God had mercy on him. And when he came near to Sara his daughter in law, he blessed her, saying, Thou art welcome, daughter: God be blessed, which hath brought thee unto us, and blessed be thy father and thy mother. And there was joy among all his brethren which were at Nineve. 18 And Achiacharus, and

Nasbas his brother's son, came: **19** And Tobias' wedding was kept seven days with great joy.

12 Raphael's secret

1 Then Tobit called his son Tobias, and said unto him, My son, see that the man have his wages, which went with thee, and thou must give him more. **2** And Tobias said unto him, O father, it is no harm to me to give him half of those things which I have brought: **3** For he hath brought me again to thee in safety, and made whole my wife, and brought me the money, and likewise healed thee. **4** Then the old man said, It is due unto him. **5** So he called the angel, and he said unto him, Take half of all that ye have brought and go away in safety.

6 Then he took them both apart, and said unto them, Bless God, praise him, and magnify him, and praise him for the things which he hath done unto you in the sight of all that live. It is good to praise God, and exalt his name, and honourably to shew forth the works of God; therefore be not slack to praise him. **7** It is good to keep close the secret of a king, but it is honourable to reveal the works of God. Do that which is good, and no evil shall touch you. **8** Prayer is good with fasting and alms and righteousness. A little with righteousness is better than much with unrighteousness. It is better to give alms than to lay up gold: **9** For alms doth deliver from death, and shall purge away all sin. Those that exercise alms and righteousness shall be filled with life:

10 But they that sin are enemies to their own life. **11** Surely I will keep close nothing from you. For I said, It was good to keep close the secret of a king, but that it was honourable to reveal the works of God. **12** Now therefore, when thou didst pray, and Sara thy daughter in law, I did bring the remembrance of your prayers before the Holy One: and when thou didst bury the dead, I was with thee likewise. **13** And when thou didst not delay to rise up, and leave thy dinner, to go and cover the dead, thy good deed was not hid from me: but I was with thee. **14** And now God hath sent me to heal thee and Sara thy daughter in law. **15** I am Raphael, one of the seven holy angels, which present the prayers of the saints, and which go in and out before the glory of the Holy One.

16 Then they were both troubled, and fell upon their faces: for they feared. **17** But he said unto them, Fear not, for it shall go well with you; praise God therefore. **18** For not of any favour of mine, but by the will of our God I came; wherefore praise him for ever. **19** All these days I did appear unto you; but I did neither eat nor drink, but ye did see a vision.

20 Now therefore give God thanks: for I go up to him that sent me; but write all things which are done in a book.

21 And when they arose, they saw him no more. **22** Then they confessed the great and wonderful works of God, and how the angel of the Lord had appeared unto them.

13 Tobit's paean of praise

1 Then Tobit wrote a prayer of rejoicing, and said, Blessed be God that liveth for ever, and blessed be his kingdom. **2** For he doth scourge, and hath mercy: he leadeth down to hell, and bringeth up again: neither is there any that can avoid his hand.

3 Confess him before the Gentiles, ye children of Israel: for he hath scattered us among them. **4** There declare his greatness, and extol him before all the living: for he is our Lord, and he is the God our Father for ever. **5** And he will scourge us for our iniquities, and will have mercy again, and will gather us out of all nations, among whom he hath scattered us.

6 If ye turn to him with your whole heart, and with your whole mind, and deal uprightly before him, then will he turn unto you, and will not hide his face from you. Therefore see what he will do with you, and confess him with your whole mouth, and praise the Lord of might, and extol the everlasting King. In the land of my captivity do I praise him, and declare his might and majesty to a sinful nation. O ye sinners, turn and do justice before him: who can tell if he will accept you, and have mercy on you? **7** I will extol my God, and my soul shall praise the King of heaven, and shall rejoice in his greatness. **8** Let all men speak, and let all praise him for his righteousness.

9 O Jerusalem, the holy city, he will scourge thee for thy children's works, and will have mercy again on the sons of the righteous. **10** Give praise to the Lord, for he is good: and praise the everlasting King, that his tabernacle may be builded in thee again with joy, and let him make joyful there in thee those that are captives, and love in thee for ever those that are miserable. **11** Many nations shall come from far to the name of the Lord God with gifts in their hands, even gifts to the King of heaven; all generations shall praise thee with great joy. **12** Cursed are all they which hate thee, and blessed shall all be which love thee for ever. **13** Rejoice and be glad for the children of the just: for they shall be gathered together, and shall bless the Lord of the just. **14** O blessed are they which love thee, for they shall rejoice in thy peace: blessed are they which have been sorrowful for all thy scourges; for they shall rejoice for thee, when they have seen all thy glory, and shall be glad for ever. **15** Let my soul bless God the great King. **16** For Jerusalem shall be built up with sapphires and emeralds, and precious stone: thy walls and towers and battlements with pure gold. **17** And the streets of Jerusalem shall be paved with beryl and carbuncle and stones of Ophir. **18** And all her streets shall say, Alleluia; and they shall praise him, saying, Blessed be God, which hath extolled it for ever.

14 The last warnings of Tobias the elder

1 So Tobit made an end of praising God. **2** And he was eight and fifty years old when he lost his sight, which was restored to him after eight years: and he gave alms, and he increased in the fear of the Lord God, and praised him. **3** And when he was very aged he called his son, and the sons of his son, and said to him, My son, take thy children; for, behold, I am aged, and am ready to depart out of this life. **4** Go into Media my son, for I surely believe those things which Jonas the prophet spake of Nineve, that it shall be overthrown; and that for a time peace shall rather be in Media; and that our brethren shall lie scattered in the earth from that good land: and Jerusalem shall be desolate, and the house of God in it shall be burned, and shall be desolate for a time; **5** And that again God will have mercy on them, and bring them again into the land, where they shall build a temple, but not like to the first, until the time of that age be fulfilled; and afterward they shall return from all places of their captivity, and build up Jerusalem gloriously, and the house of God shall be built in it for ever with a glorious building, as the prophets have spoken thereof. **6** And all nations shall turn, and fear the Lord God truly, and shall bury their idols. **7** So shall all nations praise the Lord, and his people shall confess God, and the Lord shall exalt his people; and all those which love the Lord God in truth and justice shall rejoice, shewing mercy to our brethren.

The last years of Tobit the younger

8 And now, my son, depart out of Nineve, because that those things which the prophet Jonas spake shall surely come to pass. **9** But keep thou the law and the commandments, and shew thyself merciful and just, that it may go well with thee. **10** And bury me decently, and thy mother with me; but tarry no longer at Nineve. Remember, my son, how Aman handled Achiacharus that brought him up, how out of light he brought him into darkness, and how he rewarded him again: yet Achiacharus was saved, but the other had his reward: for he went down into darkness. Manasses gave alms, and escaped the snares of death which they had set for him: but Aman fell into the snare, and perished. **11** Wherefore now, my son, consider what alms doeth, and how righteousness doth deliver. When he had said these things, he gave up the ghost in the bed, being an hundred and eight and fifty years old; and he buried him honourably. **12** And when Anna his mother was dead, he buried her with his father. But Tobias departed with his wife and children to Ecbatane to Raguel his father in law, **13** Where he became old with honour, and he buried his father and mother in law honourably, and he inherited their substance, and his father Tobit's. **14** And he died at Ecbatane in Media, being an hundred and seven and twenty years old. **15** But before he died he heard of the destruction of Nineve, which was taken by Nabuchodonosor and Assuerus: and before his death he rejoiced over Nineve.

From the Book of Job
King James Version

1

1 There was a man in the land of Uz, whose name was Job; and that man was perfect and upright, and one that feared God, and eschewed evil. **2** And there were born unto him seven sons and three daughters. **3** His substance also was seven thousand sheep, and three thousand camels, and five hundred yoke of oxen, and five hundred she asses, and a very great household; so that this man was the greatest of all the men of the east. **4** And his sons went and feasted in their houses, every one his day; and sent and called for their three sisters to eat and to drink with them. **5** And it was so, when the days of their feasting were gone about, that Job sent and sanctified them, and rose up early in the morning, and offered burnt offerings according to the number of them all: for Job said, It may be that my sons have sinned, and cursed God in their hearts. Thus did Job continually. **6** Now there was a day when the sons of God came to present themselves before the LORD, and Satan came also among them. **7** And the LORD said unto Satan, Whence comest thou? Then Satan answered the LORD, and said, From going to and fro in the earth, and from walking up and down in it. **8** And the LORD said unto Satan, Hast thou considered my servant Job, that there is none like him in the earth, a perfect and an upright man, one that feareth God, and escheweth evil? **9** Then Satan answered the LORD, and said, Doth Job fear God for nought? **10** Hast not thou made an hedge about him, and about his house, and about all that he hath on every side? thou hast blessed the work of his hands, and his substance is increased in the land. **11** But put forth thine hand now, and touch all that he hath, and he will curse thee to thy face. **12** And the LORD said unto Satan, Behold, all that he hath is in thy power; only upon himself put not forth thine hand. So Satan went forth from the presence of the LORD. **13** And there was a day when his sons and his daughters were eating and drinking wine in their eldest brother's house: **14** And there came a messenger unto Job, and said, The oxen were plowing, and the asses feeding beside them: **15** And the Sabeans fell upon them, and took them away; yea, they have slain the servants with the edge of the sword; and I only am escaped alone to tell thee. **16** While he was yet speaking, there came also another, and said, The fire of God is fallen from heaven, and hath burned up the sheep, and the servants, and consumed them; and I only am escaped alone to tell thee. **17** While he was yet speaking, there came also another, and said, The Chaldeans made out three bands, and fell upon the

camels, and have carried them away, yea, and slain the servants with the edge of the sword; and I only am escaped alone to tell thee. **18** While he was yet speaking, there came also another, and said, Thy sons and thy daughters were eating and drinking wine in their eldest brother's house: **19** And, behold, there came a great wind from the wilderness, and smote the four corners of the house, and it fell upon the young men, and they are dead; and I only am escaped alone to tell thee. **20** Then Job arose, and rent his mantle, and shaved his head, and fell down upon the ground, and worshipped, **21** And said, Naked came I out of my mother's womb, and naked shall I return thither: the LORD gave, and the LORD hath taken away; blessed be the name of the LORD. **22** In all this Job sinned not, nor charged God foolishly.

2

1 Again there was a day when the sons of God came to present themselves before the LORD, and Satan came also among them to present himself before the LORD. **2** And the LORD said unto Satan, From whence comest thou? And Satan answered the LORD, and said, From going to and fro in the earth, and from walking up and down in it. **3** And the LORD said unto Satan, Hast thou considered my servant Job, that there is none like him in the earth, a perfect and an upright man, one that feareth God, and escheweth evil? and still he holdeth fast his integrity, although thou movedst me against him, to destroy him without cause. **4** And Satan answered the LORD, and said, Skin for skin, yea, all that a man hath will he give for his life. **5** But put forth thine hand now, and touch his bone and his flesh, and he will curse thee to thy face. **6** And the LORD said unto Satan, Behold, he is in thine hand; but save his life. **7** So went Satan forth from the presence of the LORD, and smote Job with sore boils from the sole of his foot unto his crown. **8** And he took him a potsherd to scrape himself withal; and he sat down among the ashes. **9** Then said his wife unto him, Dost thou still retain thine integrity? curse God, and die. **10** But he said unto her, Thou speakest as one of the foolish women speaketh. What? shall we receive good at the hand of God, and shall we not receive evil? In all this did not Job sin with his lips. **11** Now when Job's three friends heard of all this evil that was come upon him, they came every one from his own place; Eliphaz the Temanite, and Bildad the Shuhite, and Zophar the Naamathite: for they had made an appointment together to come to mourn with him and to comfort him. **12** And when they lifted up their eyes afar off, and knew him not, they lifted up their voice, and wept; and they rent every one his mantle, and sprinkled dust upon their heads toward heaven. **13** So they sat down with him upon the ground seven days and seven nights, and none spake a word unto him: for they saw that his grief was very great.

3

1 After this opened Job his mouth, and cursed his day. **2** And Job spake, and said, **3** Let the day perish wherein I was born, and the night in which it was said, There is a man child conceived. **4** Let that day be darkness; let not God regard it from above, neither let the light shine upon it. **5** Let darkness and the shadow of death stain it; let a cloud dwell upon it; let the blackness of the day terrify it. **6** As for that night, let darkness seize upon it; let it not be joined unto the days of the year, let it not come into the number of the months. **7** Lo, let that night be solitary, let no joyful voice come therein. **8** Let them curse it that curse the day, who are ready to raise up their mourning. **9** Let the stars of the twilight thereof be dark; let it look for light, but have none; neither let it see the dawning of the day: **10** Because it shut not up the doors of my mother's womb, nor hid sorrow from mine eyes. **11** Why died I not from the womb? why did I not give up the ghost when I came out of the belly? **12** Why did the knees prevent me? or why the breasts that I should suck? **13** For now should I have lain still and been quiet, I should have slept: then had I been at rest, **14** With kings and counsellors of the earth, which built desolate places for themselves; **15** Or with princes that had gold, who filled their houses with silver: **16** Or as an hidden untimely birth I had not been; as infants which never saw light. **17** There the wicked cease from troubling; and there the weary be at rest. **18** There the prisoners rest together; they hear not the voice of the oppressor. **19** The small and great are there; and the servant is free from his master. **20** Wherefore is light given to him that is in misery, and life unto the bitter in soul; **21** Which long for death, but it cometh not; and dig for it more than for hid treasures; **22** Which rejoice exceedingly, and are glad, when they can find the grave? **23** Why is light given to a man whose way is hid, and whom God hath hedged in? **24** For my sighing cometh before I eat, and my roarings are poured out like the waters. **25** For the thing which I greatly feared is come upon me, and that which I was afraid of is come unto me. **26** I was not in safety, neither had I rest, neither was I quiet; yet trouble came.

4

1 Then Eliphaz the Temanite answered and said, **2** If we assay to commune with thee, wilt thou be grieved? but who can withhold himself from speaking? **3** Behold, thou hast instructed many, and thou hast strengthened the weak hands. **4** Thy words have upholden him that was falling, and thou hast strengthened the feeble knees. **5** But now it is come upon thee, and thou faintest; it toucheth thee, and thou art troubled. **6** Is not this thy fear, thy confidence, thy hope, and the uprightness of thy ways? **7** Remember, I pray thee, who ever perished, being innocent? or where were the righteous cut off? **8** Even as I have seen, they that plow iniquity, and sow wickedness, reap the same. **9** By the blast of God they perish, and by the breath of his nostrils are they consumed. **10** The roaring of the lion, and the voice of the fierce lion, and the teeth of the young lions, are broken. **11** The old lion perisheth for lack of prey, and the stout lion's whelps are scattered abroad. **12** Now a thing was secretly brought to me, and mine ear received a little thereof. **13** In thoughts from the visions of the night, when deep sleep falleth on men, **14** Fear came upon me, and trembling, which made all my bones to shake. **15** Then a spirit passed before my face; the hair of my flesh stood up: **16** It stood still, but I could not discern the form thereof: an image was before mine eyes, there was silence, and I heard a voice, saying, **17** Shall mortal man be more just than God? shall a man be more pure than his maker? **18** Behold, he put no trust in his servants; and his angels he charged with folly: **19** How much less in them that dwell in houses of clay, whose foundation is in the dust, which are crushed before the moth? **20** They are destroyed from morning to evening: they perish for ever without any regarding it. **21** Doth not their excellency which is in them go away? they die, even without wisdom.

5

1 Call now, if there be any that will answer thee; and to which of the saints wilt thou turn? **2** For wrath killeth the foolish man, and envy slayeth the silly one. **3** I have seen the foolish taking root: but suddenly I cursed his habitation. **4** His children are far from safety, and they are crushed in the gate, neither is there any to deliver them. **5** Whose harvest the hungry eateth up, and taketh it even out of the thorns, and the robber swalloweth up their substance. **6** Although affliction cometh not forth of the dust, neither doth trouble spring out of the ground; **7** Yet man is born unto trouble, as the sparks fly upward. **8** I would seek unto God, and unto God would I commit my cause: **9** Which doeth great things and unsearchable; marvellous things without number: **10** Who giveth rain upon the earth, and sendeth waters upon the fields: **11** To set up on high those that be low; that those which mourn may be exalted to safety. **12** He disappointeth the devices of the crafty, so that their hands cannot perform their enterprise. **13** He taketh the wise in their own craftiness: and the counsel of the froward is carried headlong. **14** They meet with darkness in the daytime, and grope in the noonday as in the night. **15** But he saveth the poor from the sword, from their mouth, and from the hand of the mighty. **16** So the poor hath hope, and iniquity stoppeth her mouth. **17** Behold, happy is the man whom God correcteth: therefore despise not thou the chastening of the Almighty: **18** For he maketh sore, and bindeth up: he woundeth, and his hands make whole. **19** He shall deliver thee in six troubles: yea, in seven there shall no evil touch thee. **20** In famine he shall redeem thee from death: and in war from the power of the sword. **21** Thou shalt be hid from the scourge of the tongue: neither shalt thou be afraid of destruction when it cometh. **22** At destruction and famine thou shalt laugh: neither shalt thou be afraid of the beasts of the earth. **23** For thou shalt be in league with the stones of the field: and the beasts of the field shall be at peace with thee. **24** And thou shalt know that thy tabernacle shall be in peace; and thou shalt visit thy habitation, and shalt not sin. **25** Thou shalt know also that thy seed shall be great, and thine offspring as the grass of the earth. **26** Thou shalt come to thy grave in a full age, like as a shock of corn cometh in in his season. **27** Lo this, we have searched it, so it is; hear it, and know thou it for thy good.

10

1 My soul is weary of my life; I will leave my complaint upon myself; I will speak in the bitterness of my soul. **2** I will say unto God, Do not condemn me; shew me wherefore thou contendest with me. **3** Is it good unto thee that thou shouldest oppress, that thou shouldest despise the work of thine hands, and shine upon the counsel of the wicked? **4** Hast thou eyes of flesh? or seest thou as man seeth? **5** Are thy days as the days of man? are thy years as man's days, **6** That thou enquirest after mine iniquity, and searchest after my sin? **7** Thou knowest that I am not wicked; and there is none that can deliver out of thine hand. **8** Thine hands have made me and fashioned me together round about; yet thou dost destroy me. **9** Remember, I beseech thee, that thou hast made me as the clay; and wilt thou bring me into dust again? **10** Hast thou not poured me out as milk, and curdled me like cheese? **11** Thou hast clothed me with skin and flesh, and hast fenced me with bones and sinews. **12** Thou hast granted me life and favour, and thy visitation hath preserved my spirit. **13** And these things hast thou hid in thine heart: I know that this is with thee. **14** If I sin, then thou markest me, and thou wilt not acquit me from mine iniquity. **15** If I be wicked, woe unto me; and if I be righteous, yet will I not lift up my head. I am full of confusion; therefore see thou mine affliction; **16** For it increaseth. Thou huntest me as a fierce lion: and again thou shewest thyself marvellous upon me. **17** Thou renewest thy witnesses against me, and increasest thine indignation upon me; changes and war are against me. **18** Wherefore then hast thou brought me forth out of the womb? Oh that I had given up the ghost, and no eye had seen me! **19** I should have been as though I had not been; I should have been carried from the womb to the grave. **20** Are not my days few? cease then, and let me alone, that I may take comfort a little, **21** Before I go whence I shall not return, even to the land of darkness and the shadow of death; **22** A land of darkness, as darkness itself; and of the shadow of death, without any order, and where the light is as darkness.

38

1 Then the LORD answered Job out of the whirlwind, and said, **2** Who is this that darkeneth counsel by words without knowledge? **3** Gird up now thy loins like a man; for I will demand of thee, and answer thou me. **4** Where wast thou when I laid the foundations of the earth? declare, if thou hast understanding. **5** Who hath laid the measures thereof, if thou knowest? or who hath stretched the line upon it? **6** Whereupon are the foundations thereof fastened? or who laid the corner stone thereof; **7** When the morning stars sang together, and all the sons of God shouted for joy? **8** Or who shut up the sea with doors, when it brake forth, as if it had issued out of the womb? **9** When I made the cloud the garment thereof, and thick darkness a swaddlingband for it, **10** And brake up for it my decreed place, and set bars and doors, **11** And said, Hitherto shalt thou come, but no further: and here shall thy proud waves be stayed? **12** Hast thou commanded the morning since thy days; and caused the dayspring to know his place; **13** That it might take hold of the ends of the earth, that the wicked might be shaken out of it? **14** It is turned as clay to the seal; and they stand as a garment. **15** And from the wicked their light is withholden, and the high arm shall be broken. **16** Hast thou entered into the springs of the sea? or hast thou walked in the search of the depth? **17** Have the gates of death been opened unto thee? or hast thou seen the doors of the shadow of death? **18** Hast thou perceived the breadth of the earth? declare if thou knowest it all. **19** Where is the way where light dwelleth? and as for darkness, where is the place thereof, **20** That thou shouldest take it to the bound thereof, and that thou shouldest know the paths to the house thereof? **21** Knowest thou it, because thou wast then born? or because the number of thy days is great? **22** Hast thou entered into the treasures of the snow? or hast thou seen the treasures of the hail, 23 Which I have reserved against the time of trouble, against the day of battle and war? 24 By what way is the light parted, which scattereth the east wind upon the earth? 25 Who hath divided a watercourse for the overflowing of waters, or a way for the lightning of thunder; 26 To cause it to rain on the earth, where no man is; on the wilderness, wherein there is no man; 27 To satisfy the desolate and waste ground; and to cause the bud of the tender herb to spring forth? 28 Hath the rain a father? or who hath begotten the drops of dew? 29 Out of whose womb came the ice? and the hoary frost of heaven, who hath gendered it? 30 The waters are hid as with a stone, and the face of the deep is frozen. 31 Canst thou bind the sweet influences of Pleiades, or loose the bands of Orion? 32 Canst thou bring forth Mazzaroth in his season? or canst thou guide Arcturus with his sons? 33 Knowest thou the ordinances of heaven? canst thou set the dominion thereof in the earth? 34 Canst thou lift up thy voice to the clouds, that abundance of waters may cover thee? 35 Canst thou send lightnings, that they may go, and say unto thee, Here we are? 36 Who hath put wisdom in the inward parts? or who hath given understanding to the heart? 37 Who can number the clouds in wisdom? or who can stay the bottles of heaven, 38 When the dust groweth into hardness, and the clods cleave fast together? 39 Wilt thou hunt the prey for the lion? or fill the appetite of the young lions, 40 When they couch in their dens, and abide in the covert to lie in wait? 41 Who provideth for the raven his food? when his young ones cry unto God, they wander for lack of meat.

42

1 Then Job answered the LORD, and said, 2 I know that thou canst do every thing, and that no thought can be withholden from thee. 3 Who is he that hideth counsel without knowledge? therefore have I uttered that I understood not; things too wonderful for me, which I knew not. 4 Hear, I beseech thee, and I will speak: I will demand of thee, and declare thou unto me. 5 I have heard of thee by the hearing of the ear: but now mine eye seeth thee. 6 Wherefore I abhor myself, and repent in dust and ashes. 7 And it was so, that after the LORD had spoken these words unto Job, the LORD said to Eliphaz the Temanite, My wrath is kindled against thee, and against thy two friends: for ye have not spoken of me the thing that is right, as my servant Job hath. 8 Therefore take unto you now seven bullocks and seven rams, and go to my servant Job, and offer up for your-selves a burnt offering; and my servant Job shall pray for you: for him will I accept: lest I deal with you after your folly, in that ye have not

spoken of me the thing which is right, like my servant Job. **9** So Eliphaz the Temanite and Bildad the Shuhite and Zophar the Naamathite went, and did according as the LORD commanded them: the LORD also accepted Job. **10** And the LORD turned the captivity of Job, when he prayed for his friends: also the LORD gave Job twice as much as he had before. **11** Then came there unto him all his brethren, and all his sisters, and all they that had been of his acquaintance before, and did eat bread with him in his house: and they bemoaned him, and comforted him over all the evil that the LORD had brought upon him: every man also gave him a piece of money, and every one an earring of gold. **12** So the LORD blessed the latter end of Job more than his beginning: for he had fourteen thousand sheep, and six thousand camels, and a thousand yoke of oxen, and a thousand she asses. **13** He had also seven sons and three daughters. **14** And he called the name of the first, Jemima; and the name of the second, Kezia; and the name of the third, Kerenhappuch. **15** And in all the land were no women found so fair as the daughters of Job: and their father gave them inheritance among their brethren. **16** After this lived Job an hundred and forty years, and saw his sons, and his sons' sons, even four generations. **17** So Job died, being old and full of days.

Invocation of Raphael by Bernard Lievegoed (1905 – 1992)

Spoken in Dutch on 16 February 1982 at the end of a lecture to prepare the laying of the foundation stone of Rafaël-Zaal in Stenia, Netherlands.

Raphael!
Brother of Humanity –
who stands beside us
giving us courage
where we healing wish to work –
where destiny run aground
we bring to evolve again.
Who redeeming,
sets aflame
the darkness of earth
in light and warmth
around his staff.
Help us –
because we also want
to change human darkness
And let human light and warmth
blaze in human hearts.

Bibliography

HANNAH ARENDT: *Eichmann in Jerusalem. A Report on the Banality of Evil.*
Penguin Classics 2010

JOHANN WOLFGANG GOETHE: *Faust.* The Harvard Classics. 1909-14

JOHANN WOLFGANG GOETHE: *The Green Snake and the Beautiful Lily,*
SteinerBooks 2006

JOHANN WOLFGANG GOETHE: *West-östlicher Divan.* Insel-Verlag 1974

MICHAELA GLÖCKLER: *Can Cancer Be Prevented?* Der Merkurstab 62:416-
420, 2009

MICHAELA GLÖCKLER (ED.): *Ethical Considerations in Medicine. Conscience,
Social Community Building, Path of Healing.* Medical Section at the
Goetheanum 2003

MICHAELA GLÖCKLER (ED.): *Meditations on Heart-Activity by Rudolf Steiner.*
Medical Section at the Goetheanum 2014

THE KING JAMES BIBLE ONLINE: *King James Bible 2015*

SILKE HELWIG: *'Es geht um mein Leben': Zum 100. Geburtstag von Rita Leroi.*
Zbinden Verlag 2013

MARGARETE AND ERICH KIRCHNER-BOCKHOLT: *Die Menschheitsaufgabe
Rudolf Steiners und Ita Wegman.* Philosophisch-Anthroposophischer Verlag
1976

MEDICAL SECTION AT THE GOETHEANUM: *Rundbrief für die Mitarbeiter der
Medizinischen Sektion am Goetheanum in aller Welt,* No. 2. Advent 1993

CHRISTIAN MORGENSTERN: *Wir fanden einen Pfad.* Zbinden Verlag 2014

CHRISTOPH RUBENS, PETER SELG (ED.): *Das menschliche Herz. Kardiologie in
der Anthroposophischen Medizin.* Ita Wegman Verlag 2014

RUDOLF STEINER: *Anthroposophical Leading Thoughts. Anthroposophy as a
Path of Knowledge. The Michael Mystery.* Rudolf Steiner Press 1999
(vol. GA 26)

RUDOLF STEINER: *The Apocalypse of St. John.* Kessinger Publishing 2010
(vol. GA 104)

RUDOLF STEINER: *Atlantis and Lemuria.* Fredonia Books 2002 (vol. GA 11)

RUDOLF STEINER: *Becoming the Archangel Michael's Companion.*
SteinerBooks 2007 (vol. GA 217)

RUDOLF STEINER: *Broken Structures. The Spiritual Structure of Human Frailty.*
Anthroposophic Press 2003 (vol. GA 318)

RUDOLF STEINER: *The Christmas Conference for the Foundation of the General
Anthroposophical Society 1923-1924.* Anthroposophic Press 1990
(vol. GA 260)

RUDOLF STEINER: *Course for Young Doctors.* Mercury Press 1997
(vol. GA 316)

RUDOLF STEINER: *Education for Special Needs. The Curative Education
Course.* Rudolf Steiner Press 1999 (vol. GA 317)

RUDOLF STEINER: *An Esoteric Cosmology*. St. George Publications 1978 (vol. GA 94)

RUDOLF STEINER: *The Fifth Gospel*. Rudolf Steiner Press 2007 (vol. GA 148)

RUDOLF STEINER: *The Four Seasons and the Archangels*. Rudolf Steiner Press 2002 (vol. GA 229)

RUDOLF STEINER: *"Freemasonry" and Ritual Work. The Misraim Service. Texts and Documents from the Cognitive-Ritual Section of the Esoteric School 1904-1919*. SteinerBooks 2007 (vol. GA 265)

RUDOLF STEINER: *From the History and Contents of the First Section of the Esoteric School 1904-1914*. SteinerBooks 2007 (vol. GA 264)

RUDOLF STEINER, ITA WEGMAN: *Fundamentals of Therapy*. Mercury Press 1999 (vol. GA 27)

RUDOLF STEINER: *How to Know Higher Worlds - A Modern Path of Initiation*. Anthroposophic Press 1994 (vol. GA 10)

RUDOLF STEINER: *Intuitive Thinking as a Spiritual Path - A Philosophy of Freedom*. Anthroposophic Press 1995 (vol. GA 4)

RUDOLF STEINER: *Manifestations of Karma*. Rudolf Steiner Press 2011 (vol. GA 120)

RUDOLF STEINER: *Mantrische Sprüche. Seelenübungen II*. 1903-1925. Rudolf Steiner Verlag 1999 (vol. GA 268)

RUDOLF STEINER: *Mystery Knowledge and Mystery Centres*. Rudolf Steiner Press 1973 (vol. GA 232)

RUDOLF STEINER: *Occult Science*. Anthroposophic Press 2009 (vol. GA 13)

RUDOLF STEINER: *Original Impulses for the Science of the Spirit*. Completion Press 2001 (vol. GA 96)

RUDOLF STEINER: *Die soziale Grundforderung unserer Zeit. In geänderter Zeitlage*. Rudolf Steiner Verlag 1990 (vol. GA 186)

RUDOLF STEINER: *Soziales Verständnis aus geisteswissenschaftlicher Erkenntnis*. Rudolf Steiner Verlag 1989 (vol. GA 191)

RUDOLF STEINER: *Verses and Meditations*. Rudolf Steiner Press 2004 (vol. GA 268)

PETER SELG: *Die "Wärme-Meditation". Geschichtlicher Hintergrund und ideelle Beziehungen*. Verlag am Goetheanum 2005

J. E. ZEYLMANS-VAN EMMICHOVEN: *Die Erkraftung des Herzens: Eine Mysterienschulung der Gegenwart. Rudolf Steiners Anleitungen für Ita Wegman*. Ita Wegman Institut 2009

J. E. ZEYLMANS-VAN EMMICHOVEN: *Who Was Ita Wegman?* vol. 2, Mercury Press 1995

www.ingramcontent.com/pod-product-compliance
Lightning Source LLC
Chambersburg PA
CBHW060643210326
41520CB00010B/1722